To Get Back Home

To Get Back Home

◆

A Mysterious Disease: A Fight for Life

Wendy Chapin Ford

iUniverse, Inc.
New York Bloomington

Copyright © 2009 by Wendy Chapin Ford

All rights reserved. No part of this book may be used or reproduced by any means, graphic, electronic, or mechanical, including photocopying, recording, taping or by any information storage retrieval system without the written permission of the publisher except in the case of brief quotations embodied in critical articles and reviews.

iUniverse books may be ordered through booksellers or by contacting:

iUniverse
1663 Liberty Drive
Bloomington, IN 47403
www.iuniverse.com
1-800-Authors (1-800-288-4677)

Because of the dynamic nature of the Internet, any Web addresses or links contained in this book may have changed since publication and may no longer be valid. The views expressed in this work are solely those of the author and do not necessarily reflect the views of the publisher, and the publisher hereby disclaims any responsibility for them.

ISBN: 978-1-4401-9916-5 (sc)
ISBN: 978-1-4401-9914-1 (dj)
ISBN: 978-1-4401-9915-8 (ebook)

Printed in the United States of America

iUniverse rev. date: 01/08/10

For Westy and Lindsay,

my great motivation

and

for B.G.,

our shooting star

Nothing in life is as exhilarating as to be shot at without result.

—Winston Churchill

"Acute disseminating encephalomyelitis (ADEM) is an acute or subacute illness that typically follows a viral infection or immunization. Pathologically, the lesions of ADEM are areas of demyelination. Demyelination refers to the destruction of some or all of the myelin sheath. Myelin insulates the nerve axon. In ADEM, normally it is destroyed by the body's immune system because the system is no longer capable of recognizing the myelin as belonging to the self, rather as a foreign invader that must be destroyed.

"The typical clinical presentation of ADEM is multifocal neurologic abnormalities reflecting a widespread central nervous system disturbance.

"Neurologic symptoms in ADEM characteristically begin one to three weeks after an infection or immunization. The illness has been described following rubeola, vaccinia, varicella, mycoplasma, mumps, rubella, and nonspecific respiratory infections, but may occur without a recognizable preceding event ... Confusion and lethargy are frequent and may progress to coma ..."

—Adapted from "MRI in acute disseminated encephalomyelitis"
by K. S. Caldemeyer, R. R. Smith, T. M. Harris, M. K. Edwards.
Neuro-radiology Springer-Verlag, 1994

Contents

Part One
Chapter One: *B.G., I can't walk!* 1

Chapter Two: To Beth Israel 5

Chapter Three: The Awakening 50

Part Two
Chapter Four: Out of the Fire 71

Chapter Five: Impossible Memories 75

Chapter Six: Pleasant, but Confused 79

Chapter Seven: To Get Back Home 84

Part Three
Chapter Eight: In Search of Meaning 135

Chapter Nine: Prayer 143

Epilogue One 153

Epilogue Two 155

My Magnificent Hospitals 157

Photographs 158

Acknowledgments 159

Notes 161

About the Cover Art 165

Part One

"Poor typist, will call. Can,t believe your alive."

e-mail from Dr. David Trentham, March 1999
Beth Israel-Deaconess Medical Center
Boston, Massachusetts

Chapter One

"B.G., I can't walk!"

On Friday evening, May 15, 1998, I enjoyed supper with my family in the seaside garden of our home on the North Shore of Boston. My husband, Bruce (a.k.a., B.G.), and I had lived there for ten years.

After spending the day in Boston, we had been determined to put some unpleasant business behind us during a delightful al fresco lunch at Maison Robert, our favorite restaurant in the city. The weather was beautiful, a clear sunny day in spring with enough warmth to hint of summer, our favorite season, which was just around the corner.

That evening back at our old colonial home, we enjoyed the warm spring breezes as our two young children, Westy and Lindsay, frolicked in the garden. Watching the sailboats in the outer harbor, we laughed and talked as we looked forward to another summer of sailing and tennis in Massachusetts and Maine. B.G. and I had sailed together for years, beginning before we were married. But it was always fresh—a time to appreciate life and reconnect. I never tired of seeing Bruce's piercing blue eyes against the backdrop of the sea. On the water, it seemed as though we were always smiling. It was ever so beautiful, and we felt so alive out there in the elements. Then, of course, we brought the children into it, and they, too, developed a love of sailing and the sea.

In the end, I remember feeling very lucky that day. The children were happy and healthy. They were at a wonderful school right in our neighborhood. We seemed to have the best of everything: good health, a beautiful family, great friends, and a charming home in a lovely town, just up the road from our favorite city. From every perspective, it seemed like a charmed life. From every perspective but one.

The memories of that evening were the last I would have for more than three weeks.

I have pieced together a chronicle of this time by drawing upon conversations and correspondence with the people who endured this ordeal with me. At times, their words help me tell the story.

♦ ♦ ♦

I awoke the next morning, Saturday, May 16, feeling ill. Both Bruce and I thought it was simply a case of the flu.

"B.G.," I said weakly, "you have to take the children out today and let me rest. I'm exhausted." He looked in on me, guessed I was coming down with nothing more than an unusually bad cold or flu, gathered Westy and Lindsay, and left for a long walk at an old estate in town. The park was beautiful that time of year, with the azaleas in bloom and the garden's famed rhododendrons starting to come out. It was a favorite destination for the whole family, and Bruce and the kids had a wonderful day.

Meanwhile, I spent the entire weekend resting. I don't remember getting out of bed at all, although I later learned that I did—even drove myself to the local hospital for some medicine. By Sunday evening, I was confused and on the verge of delirium.

Bruce had become increasingly concerned as the hours passed and I seemed to be slipping into myself. Finally, he announced, "This is no ordinary flu. If you're not better tomorrow, I'm taking you to the hospital."

By Monday morning, I was definitely not better. Bruce dressed for work, and our children's nanny, Jeanne, arrived. Westy, our seven-year-old son, was up and getting ready for school. Lindsay, our three-year-old daughter, was still asleep and thus was spared the sight of what came next.

"Wendy, you'll have to get dressed," said Bruce. "I'm taking you to the hospital."

"Okay," I said weakly, as I struggled to sit up in bed. But then a frightening problem presented itself.

"B.G.," I said, attempting to get my clothes, "I can't walk!"

Stunned, he stared at me. "You can't walk?"

"No."

He helped me dress. I had always been athletic, deriving great pleasure from sailing, skiing, playing tennis, and being outdoors. Now my muscular legs were of no use to me. He slipped them into a pair of jeans.

"Can you hand me Dad's belt?" I asked.

Lying down, I was able to loop my late father's old ostrich-skin belt, which I treasured, through my jeans. Bruce quickly picked me up, put me over his shoulders like a sack of potatoes, and carried me down the stairs.

Westy stood in the front hall, watching with his nanny, Jeanne. Both looked extremely puzzled.

Bruce carried me out of the house. I'm told it was a clear, bright morning, the kind when the sun sparkles on the harbor so beautifully, but I don't remember that. Bruce put me in the Buick station wagon, which we had owned for four years. He later told me that I looked at it and asked, "Is this a new car, B.G.?"

Staving off his concerns, Bruce drove to the fine community hospital in the center of town. He stayed with me in the emergency room as physicians examined me, gave me a spinal tap, and kept me for observation. I remember nothing.

"You'll be fine now," Bruce assured me, though undoubtedly, he had a hard time watching the clinical proceedings. "I'll check in later on, when I get to work."

Bruce left the hospital, confident that I was in capable hands. He genuinely felt that what I needed was expert attention, which he could see I was receiving. I apparently had the presence of mind to ask for, and was admitted to, a private room.

Medical Record May 18, 1998

> Patient returned to emergency room [where I had checked in over the weekend for a stubborn sinus infection, but did not recall it] with progressive headaches, confusion, neck stiffness, leg stiffness, inability to walk. Temperature 103. Lumbar Puncture performed, 620W [white blood cells, indicating infection] ... Neurologist suggests brain stem dysfunction ... Advised to Beth Israel-Deaconess Medical Center.
>
> —(unsigned)

I made two phone calls from the hospital that morning to my two closest colleagues and dear friends at John Hancock. Foster Aborn was the company's boyish but exacting vice chairman and chief investment officer. Tim Hollingworth and I had worked as financial writers side-by-side for a decade. Neither was in when I made my calls. However, once they arrived at their offices atop the gleaming, blue glass Hancock Tower overlooking Boston that morning, they found some bizarre messages waiting for them in their voice mail.

I had been Foster's speechwriter for more than a decade, but because of his demanding schedule, I always avoided taking up his time unnecessarily.

Why I would have called him when we were not working on a project at the time is puzzling. I can only guess that I must have been frightened, perhaps even terrified, given what had begun to happen. But his empathy and devotion would prove instrumental in saving my life.

"Foster ... Tim ... it's Wendy," I began slowly. My speech already showed signs of dysfunction. "I'm in the hhhhhospital. They don't nnnnknow whhhhhat's wrong, and ... I'm not sssssure when I'll be back to the office."

I rambled on, slurring my words.

Tim and Foster later expressed to me equal amounts of concern and confusion about my messages. Tim recalled thinking I sounded drunk.

In retrospect, the reason I had no memory, the reason I sounded so odd, was clear: my body had begun to shut down.

I was dying.

Chapter Two

To Beth Israel

By the next morning, it was apparent to the staff at the local hospital that my problem, still unidentified, had become fairly serious. Without hesitation, Bruce made the decision to transfer me to Boston's Beth Israel-Deaconess Medical Center (BIDMC). This Harvard Medical School teaching hospital was known as "Harvard with a Heart." We had always thought the world of Beth Israel. Our children were born there, and Bruce and I had received our medical care there for years.

It would prove to be a critical decision.

Bruce preceded the ambulance to Boston. When we arrived, I cheerfully said, "B.G., you have to meet these nice guys who drove me down!"

I was lucid and sociable; I was also failing all of the tests for strength and coordination the emergency room doctors were giving me. Each time I failed to answer a question or follow an instruction correctly, the doctors stopped and looked at each other, their eyes locked in consternation. Bruce watched with mounting concern. He quickly realized that everything was not going to be all right.

I was placed in the Medical Intensive Care Unit (MICU) where Dr. Dori Zaleznik, an infectious disease specialist, launched a therapy of antibiotics and antiviral drugs. From the beginning, Bruce referred to Dr. Zaleznik as the Pied Piper of the intensive care unit. "She moved around with about a half-dozen residents hanging on her every word," he later recalled. "If she moved left, they moved left; if she moved right ..."

After a time, Bruce asked Dr. Zaleznik what antibiotics I was being given.

Her cryptic answer: "All of them."

Thus began the roller-coaster ride, which was all downhill from the start. Bruce was now more certain than ever that I didn't have the flu, or anything remotely resembling it.

The doctors at the local hospital were very good, but I felt much better after we were settled in at Beth Israel—the big hospital—in Boston. I thought they would know exactly what to do.

—Bruce

Bruce was not a worrier by nature and moved through life with relative ease, always on an even keel. He had such confidence in Beth Israel and so expected me to be treated for this odd malady, whatever it was, and sent home within a couple of days. When he returned home to the children and went to sleep that evening, he could not have come close to guessing what had begun to play out at Beth Israel-Deaconess Medical Center with his wife of twenty-one years and mother of his two young children.

Record, Beth Israel-Deaconess

May 20, 1998

2:40 AM Radiology. Examination requested by Dr. Heather S. Harrell. Reasons for this examination:

Forty-two-year-old previously healthy woman with rapidly progressive lower extremities weakness, bowel and bladder dysfunction, sensory loss to mid-thoracic level, diplopia [a sight disorder, usually double vision], and somnolence. Evaluation for lesion in brain stem and cord.

And there was also this report, following an MRI (magnetic resonance imagery) of my brain and spinal cord:

Medical Record, Beth Israel-Deaconess

May 20, 1998

Radiology. Findings:

The brain parenchyma [tissue] is normal appearing. There is no evidence of increased T2 signal to suggest brain edema.[1] No midline shift or mass effect is present. The ventricles are patent and symmetric. There is slight increase in T2 signal in the region of the bilateral cortical spinal tracts, which is less evident on the proton density-weighted sequences. This is felt to represent a normal finding ... There is no leptomeningeal enhancement seen to suggest encephalitis. There is specifically no feature suggestive of herpes encephalitis. From the MRI of the thoracic spine, there is mild diffuse enlargement of the thoracic cord from the T1 level inferiorly with areas of high T2 signal in the cord that extend down to the conus. No contrast enhancement is seen in this region. The adjacent vertebrae are all normal appearing. From the MRI of the lumbar spine, again, areas of increased T2 signal are seen in the region of the conus. The remainder of the lumbosacral spine is unremarkable. No focal enhancing lesions are seen ...

—S. Voss, MD

—J.N. Suojanen, MD

These initial scans of my brain and spinal cord showed nothing out of the ordinary. But just a few hours later, in the waking hours of Wednesday, May 20, the alarms sounded in earnest.

Medical Record, Beth Israel-Deaconess

May 20, 1998

Intensive Care Attending, admit note:

Patient seen and examined on morning rounds. Forty-two-year-old previously well female is somnolent but arousable; falls back quickly to sleep ... There is progressive neurologic decline with possible viral illness with features of brain stem and spinal cord involvement ... No clear diagnosis at this point ... There are concerns about infectious meningitis and most likely encephalomyelitis, given extensive findings ... Would appreciate input from neurology and infectious diseases services. Will continue broad spectrum antiviral/ antibacterial coverage.

—H. Harrell, M.D.

Later that morning, Bruce received a phone call at the Chelmsford High School, in the western suburb of Boston, where he taught physics. It was the hospital, and the news was far from good. It was the first time Bruce lost hope of any possibility that I would be better anytime soon. A colleague standing near him in the teachers' lounge took one look at his face as he finished the call in disbelief, thrust her cell phone in his hand, and told him to take it and go—that they would take care of everything with his students and classes *but to just go now.*

"Mr. Ford, your wife appears to have a serious problem of a neurological nature," said Dr. Heather Harrell, an emergency room physician at Beth Israel-Deaconess. "She is going to need a neurologist."

Not surprisingly, we did not have a neurologist. Bruce always knew what to do, so, naturally, he immediately called my primary care physician of twenty years, whom I choose to call "Dr. Doolittle." She would be the only medical person who failed us through this entire episode. Bruce clearly explained the situation to her.

"Wendy is seriously ill—perhaps dangerously ill," he began. "The doctors don't know what it is, but the disorder appears to have a neurological aspect. We need the best neurologist and the best infectious disease specialist that you can possibly get—and soon."

"Well," said Dr. Doolittle, "I will probably be going over to Beth Israel later in the day. I'll try to get back to you sometime in the afternoon."

It was immediately apparent to my concerned husband that my long-time physician, who was presumably well connected to our favorite hospital, would be of little immediate help.

Stunned at her response and lack of diligence, Bruce immediately called Foster at John Hancock before even putting down the phone, his adrenaline starting to kick in. He needed action and responsiveness. Bruce would have called him regardless of Dr. Doolittle's cavalier attitude, because Foster was a trustee of the Beth Israel-Deaconess Medical Center. But his immediate response and willingness to do whatever he could to help was crucial. He had always been a steadfast, devoted friend, and Bruce knew he could count on him.

"I had no luck with Wendy's doctor," Bruce explained to Foster. "If you can make contact with a good neurologist, that is what we need. If you can't, please call me back right away."

Foster told him he would see what he could do.

◆   ◆   ◆

Foster didn't have to call back. At his request, Dr. Clifford Saper, the neurologist-in-chief of Beth Israel-Deaconess and chairman of the department of neurology at Harvard Medical School, became involved in my case at the very start. If Bruce was becoming the general in this war, then Foster was our secret agent. To complete the analogy, our sharpshooter was Dr. Thomas Scammell, a tenacious young research doctor and Harvard Medical School professor who would be named to head my neurology team.

By 1:00 PM that day, Wednesday, May 20, Dr. Saper was at my bedside. He made a handwritten entry to continue what would become a voluminous medical record.

Medical Record, Beth Israel-Deaconess

May 20, 1998

1:00 PM Neuro Chief:

Asked to see patient by family. Findings are as described by Dr. Scammell. She is arousable very briefly to voice, incoherent. Cannot follow commands ... I agree with diagnosis of infectious encephalomyelitis [and] would proceed rapidly with MRI of head and spinal cord to rule out lesion that precludes lumbar puncture [a spinal tap] and if there is more [evidence of lesions], proceed with lumbar puncture here ASAP ...

—C. Saper, MD

"Normally, a patient isn't seen by two neurologists in one day," Dr. Scammell later recalled. "But Foster called out all the troops, and Dr. Saper gave me the heads-up. We started the examination. The critical issues were the decreasing mental status, paralysis, and fever. Because of the fever and the results of the lumbar puncture, we first thought of an acute infection, such as bacterial meningitis."[2, 3]

♦ ♦ ♦

When I arrived at Beth Israel, I was lethargic, groggy, and could only follow simple commands, such as opening my eyes. Anything more complex was impossible. Already, there was poor sensation in my legs, which were flaccid (limp). I had trouble moving my eyes. My arms were weakening.

"The softness of the leg tissue indicated immediately that there was substantial spinal cord injury," Dr. Scammell explained to me months later.

10   To Get Back Home

Dr. Zaleznik, the infectious disease specialist, made a stunning entry into the medical record that first day at Beth Israel-Deaconess, one that, when I was later able to read it, shook me to the core.

Medical Record, Beth Israel-Deaconess

May 20, 1998

Infectious Diseases Attending:

Asked by Dr. Scammell to comment on possible etiology [underlying cause] and treatment for confusion, somnolence, fever, and CSF pleocytosis [elevated amount of white blood cells in the cerebral spinal fluid] in a forty-two-year-old female. Patient seen and examined. History reviewed in detail ... Also spoke at length with patient's husband ... The patient had apparently been working avidly in her garden recently and developed headache and sore throat on May 13. She was ... first given Sudafed, then Keflex, but she became confused prior to admission elsewhere and then transferred here. Her husband says there has been no appreciable travel outside of New England. They have gone to Plum Island with their children recently. No pets. He states she has been eating foods from a health store but denies supplements or alternative medicine. He notes she asked if they had a new car when driving to hospital ... Unable to say where she lives *or if she has children.* Answers yes/no questions, but not extremely accurately.

Assessment/suggestions:

This is a confusing case with exam suggestive of encephalitis, but MRIs findings suggesting myelitis ... Noninfectious etiologies are possible [but] for now would concentrate on infectious ...

—D. Zaleznik, MD

♦ ♦ ♦

Judy Atterstrom stopped in midstride. She put down the forms she had been holding onto and stared at the inert shape on the bed. Her new patient, a mother of two young children, had been wheeled in with nearly all her systems already shutting down. The patient's husband was admittedly more distraught than he ever had been in his life. An intensive care nurse for eighteen years, Judy faltered.

There, in Room Number One of the intensive care unit at Beth Israel-Deaconess, "the Ritz of Boston hospitals," Judy had begun to fill out the forms to sign on as my primary nurse. She looked at me lying in bed motionless. Like the friends and family who saw me early on, she had been struck by how very still I was. As Foster would later put it, "as though awaiting only a shroud."

> *I rarely hesitate. I've been doing this type of work for so long, but sometimes I just have to look inward and assess my ability to take on certain cases.*
>
> *I started to sign in, but I just had to stop and think. Here is a young woman, with two young children, and in very bad shape. It's not at all clear if she'll make it. I just wasn't sure if I could handle it. Some cases are like that. I don't hesitate very often, but I thought this one might be a real emotional wringer. I just went off by myself to think and try to figure out if I was up to it. In the end, I signed on because I realized that if I didn't do it, someone else would—a certain nurse on staff who was good, but single. Like Wendy, I had young children, and I thought, "I can do better. I'll be able to relate to her better."*
>
> —J. A. Atterstrom, RN

Judy wandered the corridors of the hospital for half an hour before returning to my room. She took another look at her unfortunate patient—and a couple of deep breaths—before proceeding to complete the forms to become my primary nurse. She impressed everyone who visited me in the intensive care unit as not only the most caring of nurses, but someone who actually managed my care, working tirelessly to keep me alive so that I might get better.

Keeping me alive was Judy's business, and she was the best of CEOs. Her care and management were crucial. A great portion of the medical story for cases such as mine is in the maintenance and monitoring of basic physical functions so life can simply continue. To make sure I didn't stop breathing, Judy and her team saw that my airways remained clear and open, that my tongue didn't fall back. I was suctioned frequently so that secretions wouldn't choke me or cause pneumonia. Judy and the other nurses checked me continuously for high fevers that could lead to seizures. They were ever on the lookout for infections and worked diligently to fight them.

These round-the-clock procedures, day after day and week after week, might have seemed routine. But they were critical. If Judy and her troops in intensive care had been average in any way, crucial medical intervention and treatment might not have mattered. But Judy and the other nurses on the front lines with her were Beth Israel Deaconess nurses—often referred to as national legends.

And to Judy Atterstrom, my husband, Bruce, was "Magnum, P.I."

Bruce seemed to uncover something new every day. He researched and investigated tirelessly, whether the task was to find an account of a similar malady, track down a doctor in another part of the country who had had success in treating the comatose, or look into what I had eaten for lunch at Maison Robert on May 15. Being a scientist, research was a natural activity for him and one that also probably provided a kind of refuge. Being active and constructive in that way undoubtedly helped him keep his increasing fear and worry at bay.

Bruce later admitted that he went to pieces in those first few days. Six foot one and normally strong and vibrant—a larger than life figure to so many—he was now having trouble getting his tall, muscular frame out of bed. But he quickly figured out what he had to do—get in gear. According to Foster, Bruce got himself a mission: he was prepared to move heaven and earth.

Bruce likened this episode to a war, involving literally hundreds of people, each doing his or her part. Each individual effort was crucial. But he was the general.

Judy thought Bruce's advocacy invaluable.

"What he did was very difficult," she explained. "It's easy for people in a situation like that to be obnoxious, at worst, or counterproductive. He had such a nice way about him—the way he offered the information he gathered, the findings he uncovered—always waiting for just the right moment."

When Judy told me this about Bruce, I was not at all surprised. I had often seen this kind of grace in him in the face of discomfort or potential conflict. He was always so competent, in control, and thoughtful. He just didn't make mistakes.

◆ ◆ ◆

When doctors can't identify a problem, they name a syndrome. My syndrome initially was called *meningoencephalomyelitis*, referring to an inflammation of the membrane that surrounds the brain and spinal cord. The doctors began by considering different bacteria and viruses.

Medical Record, Beth Israel-Deaconess

May 20, 1998

6:00 PM Neurology Consultant Attending:

Have examined patient again: still opens eyes to voice, doesn't know husband's name ... very weak in legs but slight perception and withdrawal to pain in feet.

Impression: meningoencephalomyelitis. Difficult diagnosis basically unchanged, but would appreciate infectious diseases input and coverage of rickettsia.[4] Today's lumbar puncture encouraging, suggests that she is moving more toward chronic phase of viral process. We considered tuberculosis or acute disseminated encephalomyelitis but both seem unlikely on history and lab findings ...

—T. Scammell, MD

For several days, the doctors suspected the nature of my disease to be infectious. Because of the aggressiveness of the disorder and my accelerated deterioration, they were particularly concerned with the possibility of Eastern equine encephalitis, which is nearly always fatal. It is unusual for someone to get so sick so fast. With the location of our home in close proximity to the beaches and famed horse country of Boston's North Shore, Lyme disease was another consideration.

Dr. Scammell called Bruce at home to ask about ticks. The doctor and his colleagues were trying to determine what sort of infection I might have. They had medicines that were very good at treating infections; they hoped they could identify this one quickly.

The antibiotic and antiviral therapy that Dr. Zaleznik ordered was continued for several days, but with no appreciable result. An MRI administered at 2:00 AM on May 20 showed that the brain was normal—although there were subtle indications of a slight inflammation of the spinal cord. The radiologists reported that a demyelinating process, which would indicate possible brain and spinal cord disorder, could give that appearance. But it easily could have been caused by an infection.

What was initially referred to as the differential diagnosis focused on two potential issues. The primary considerations were whether I had a viral or bacterial meningitis or if I had a demyelinating disease. Whatever the cause, the doctors decided to examine the MRI again due to my rapid deterioration. In addition, my confusion and fevers prompted a concern about seizures, so an electroencephalogram (EEG) was ordered as well.

"The EEG on May 21 showed slowed brain waves," Dr. Scammell explained. "Functions of your brain were becoming progressively more impaired."

Gradually, I drifted off and ultimately lost consciousness. I had become comatose.

Bruce quickly learned that medical people didn't use the word *coma* in conversation. They seemed to prefer being more specific. Or perhaps the reference was simply too frightening. But that was what happened: coma. I was alive, but just barely. Already, I had gone to another place.

And I remember nothing.

Medical Record, Beth Israel-Deaconess

May 21, 1998

6:49 AM Intensive Care, progress note:

Patient more lethargic this morning, often needing to be called two or three times before she arouses. Often doesn't answer questions, and, when she does, the answers are inappropriate. Frequently repeats words and short phrases to answer several different questions. Not moving lower extremities at all; upper extremities move weakly. Groans with turning, etc., and definitely responds to painful stimuli [for example, blood draws]. PERL [neuro exam measure indicating pupils equal and reactive to light and accommodation] varying in size. Not oriented at all .... Having brief episodes of apnea [partial suspension of breath], during which heart rate drops to 50s. Episodes are increasing in frequency.

Assessment: Continued deterioration in neurologic status.

Prognosis: Continue to closely follow. Assess for potential need for intubation and airway protection.

—(unsigned)

7:00 AM Intensive Care, progress note:

Coping: Family will be adequately supported. Family will understand treatment and plan. Have spoken to and updated patient's husband and her sister-in-law, Terri, who is a nurse. They are understandably upset and frustrated at her continued deterioration and a lack of concrete answers.

—E. F. Paradise, RN

4:59 PM Intensive Care, progress note, Neurology status:

[Patient] occasionally opens eyes to voice and to painful stimuli; no verbal response other than moaning and groaning with painful stimuli. Unable to obey commands. No spontaneous movements of lower extremities; occasionally moves left arm but is very stiff, no movement noted in right arm. PERL has episodes of restlessness, shaking head back and forth. No seizure activity noted. Neurology consult team remains involved. No new culture results, covering for bacterial and viral infection. Husband was in this morning and discussed patient's condition with the neurology consultant and the infectious disease consultant. Appears appropriately concerned. Patient's other sister-in-law and mother from out-of-state will be in this evening.

—(unsigned)

My mother, Roberta "Billie" Chapin, flew in from Michigan the day I slipped into the coma. A vibrant, cheerful 77-year-old, my mother was active and popular in our hometown of Bay City, Michigan, where she still played tennis several times a week. She impressed everyone with her youthfulness and charm, but most of all, with her positive attitude against all odds.

When she arrived on May 22, I was deeply unresponsive and nearly fully comatose.

When I received Bruce's call, I felt as though I had forgotten to breathe for the moment. Mothers always fear the day when the news from their children is bad. My being so far away made it worse.

—Billie Chapin

16   To Get Back Home

Medical Record, Beth Israel-Deaconess

May 22, 1998

5:47 AM Intensive Care, progress note:

Neuromuscular weakness: Half-hour neurology checks, with improvement noted with regard to gag and cough. Extreme weakness remains undaunted, and certainly no worse than 8:00 PM assessment. No lower extremities movement, only left upper extremity moves, with pain; right upper extremity no movement. Have been chasing fever all night. Temperature maximum 102.5 at 8:00 PM.

—J. Crivell, RN

2:45 PM Intensive Care, progress note:

Worsening neurology status. [There is] increased unresponsiveness. Only responded to pain this morning, whereas yesterday was able to open eyes and focus when name was called. Lower extremities remain unresponsive. No movement noted from right upper extremity, left arm noted for decreased unresponsiveness, unable to obey commands, and no spontaneous movements were noted. No gag reflex and impaired cough reflex noted. [Patient] was unable to handle secretions. Decision made to intubate for airway protection. Neurology doctor assessed, and also noted worsening responsiveness. [Scheduled] to repeat head and spine MRI this evening. At present, does open eyes to voice, but no other changes noted.

Coping: Family will be adequately supported. Husband called in morning before intubation. Husband and mother in to visit and were appropriately upset and very concerned. They met with intensive care doctors and with neurology consulting doctor.

—P.A. Chabre, RN

After arriving at Logan Airport, I took a cab to Beth Israel. When I walked into your room, I could hardly believe what I saw. You were unable to communicate, and you were so still. At that point, I felt as if I had left my body and was watching the scene from another dimension.

—Billie Chapin

Earlier that day, an anesthesiologist had intubated me, a sight neither Mom nor Bruce had yet seen. He placed an endotracheal tube in my nose that passed through my trachea into my lungs. It was attached to a respirator—also known as a ventilator or "vent." I also had acquired a feeding tube. While it was possible in these circumstances to feed me with intravenous nutrition, it was better to use the tube, or "gut," because it greatly reduced the chance of infection. Also, a patient is less prone to developing cholycystis, the inflammation of the gall bladder. This tube went through my mouth and into my stomach. Thus, there were tubes going into my nose and mouth, with tape over my face to hold them in place.

> *The moment Bruce saw you that way, he just turned heel and walked out into the hall. I found him, his head in his hands and near tears. I felt so very sorry for him. I sat on the arm of his chair and cradled his head in my arms. I told him things would be all right. That seemed to be my role: to be comforting and to pass the Kleenex.*
>
> —Billie Chapin

> *I knew what the tubes were for. It wasn't the sight as much as what it all meant. It meant things weren't getting better—they weren't even staying the same.*
>
> —Bruce

From the beginning, Mother's strength of spirit, optimism, and spunk stood her in great stead. It also allowed her to help others. Privately, Bruce considered her attitude illogical. Mom was in fact both logical and intelligent, but her optimism undoubtedly flew too much in the face of reality for him—the reality he had been living with for a number of days at that point. But, of course, he allowed it, and privately he understood that it was her way of coping.

In fact, things were getting worse.

Mom tried talking to me. "Wendy, dear," she said. "This has to be only a temporary thing. You'll soon be okay."

When I didn't respond, she said, "Can you open your eyes, 'Poo?'"

No response.

"Can you move your fingers?"

No response.

> *It was very hard to accept your condition. Bruce and I found it so hard to see you in that comatose state, with the tubes and your labored*

breathing sounds. I kept telling myself that you would get through this. The situation brought me back to when I lost your father. I wanted to cry, but I just couldn't. It was as if someone had short-circuited my emotional wires. I was just waiting for the switch to be turned on again.

Someone said I must have had ice-water in my veins, but that was not so. I just couldn't give in to the sadness I really felt, and I suppose it made me feel better for it.

—Billie Chapin

♦ ♦ ♦

Medical Record, Beth Israel-Deaconess

May 22, 1998

5:02 PM Internal Medicine, progress note:

[Patient] remains minimally responsive, withdraws/grimaces to pain ... responds to noxious stimuli, but not to voice [and] unable to cooperate with neuro exam. [She] remains significantly debilitated, with stable cognitive impairment, perhaps some continued worsening of lower extremities motor function ... Fevers persist ... Tolerating tube feeds ... Progressive worsening of delirium. Now on ventilator ... Follow respiratory status for evidence of superimposed bacterial process.

—(unsigned)

Neurology Consultant Attending:

Nearly comatose, opens eyes spontaneously to sound on occasion but usually needs more vigorous stimuli ... EEG shows slowing; other labs unchanged ... Awaiting results of repeat MRI ... Repeat EEG tomorrow to rule out the unlikely possibility of nonconvulsive seizures.

—T. Scammell, MD

There was very little hope for me at Beth Israel-Deaconess during this time. There was neither optimism nor any statement that even remotely suggested a positive outcome.

"The seriousness of the situation made it extremely difficult for anyone to say anything hopeful," Dr. Scammell later confessed. "The situation was very grim."

With nothing to communicate, the doctors simply shook their heads and looked grave. They knew better than anyone that raising false hopes might ultimately be cruel. Still, their message could not have been clearer to Bruce. A fatal outcome seemed very much in the offing.

> *I would wake up in the middle of the night and think, at first, that it had all been a nightmare. Then the reality would hit. The house was so quiet, except for the sounds of Lindsay stirring, over the intercom. Then I would remember the hospital and realize I was living a nightmare. The doctors looked the way they would if they were handing you a sympathy card. It was impossible not to understand.*
>
> —Bruce

One resident deigned to comment. "There's a fifty-fifty chance she'll make it," he told Bruce. While Bruce thought the young doctor had probably spoken out of school, the odds were better than what he had been imagining, so he took some ironic comfort from those numbers. From the doctor's statement he was able to absorb, for the first time, the possibility that the situation might be better than he had been thinking, that his wife might not die. He was able to latch on to this other possibility, and it gave him hope he hadn't had before.

But there I was, at one of the greatest hospitals in the world, receiving the best possible care. The most impressive resources and attention were directed toward my case. Doctors and researchers continued to search valiantly and diligently to determine what should be done. But the medical mystery persisted. As hard as they tried, none of the doctors, from their wide range of specialties, could make a diagnosis. And without a diagnosis, they could not initiate a treatment. All the Beth Israel-Deac's horses and all the Beth Israel-Deac's men and women simply could not figure out how to put me back together again. Meanwhile, almost by the hour, I was slipping toward the abyss.

According to Dr. Scammell, the intensive care staff was very agitated by this case of a previously healthy woman who had become so sick so suddenly.

Room One at Beth Israel-Deaconess Medical Intensive Care Unit was an especially busy and discouraging place in May 1998.

Medical Record, Beth Israel-Deaconess

May 23, 1998

3:51 AM Intensive Care, progress note:

No bilateral lower extremity movement, no movement to right upper extremity and notably less movement to left upper extremity.

Please note: developing foot drop [and] needs buck boots as soon as possible from occupational therapy ... No spontaneous or provoked eye opening. [Patient] remains febrile [feverish] ... Temperature hovering in the 100s last night.

—J. Crivell, RN

3:40 PM Progress note:

Minimal change, remains deeply comatose. Discussed utility of empiric steroids and brain biopsy potentially more dangerous than helpful without clear abnormality on imaging studies ... Steroids similarly risky, given continued belief that the primary process is likely infectious ... If cultures remain negative and lumbar probe suggests worsening inflammation and clinical course remains poor, will have more justification to start steroids.

—M. G. McLaughlin, MD

Neurology Attending:

Patient examined. Does not open eyes to command; minimal grimacing to pain; no withdrawal of right upper extremity to pain; minimal motion of left upper extremity to pain; no withdrawal of either lower extremity. Pupils unequal, left slightly larger than right.

—(signature illegible)

5:21 PM Progress note:

All questions (steroids, brain biopsy) answered to husband's satisfaction. He would like to speak with a social worker regarding therapy for his children… Subject of tracheostomy, PEG [a feeding tube inserted directly into the stomach], and long rehabilitation introduced.

—J. A. Atterstrom, RN

◆ ◆ ◆

I began to prepare myself for three different outcomes. The first and most obvious one was death. The second was survival, if and when the doctors could make a diagnosis and initiate treatment. Then, the question came to revolve around the extent of recovery. If it happened, would it be partial, physically or cognitively? The third possibility, which I had been given no logical reason to hope for, was complete recovery.

But for that, it seemed like a miracle would have to occur.

—Bruce

Our daughter Lindsay, barely three years old, could not possibly have understood the reason for her mother's sudden, extended absence. One night, I was reading her bedtime stories and singing lullabies; the next day, I was gone. My son Westy, nearly eight, understood only that his mom was in the hospital and doctors were working hard to make her better. Although many friends, relatives, and nannies stepped into the breach to help with the children, this period of time meant a tortuous psychological balancing act for Bruce.

What he couldn't do was tell the children when—or even if—their mother would be coming home. There was a very long period when it was not apparent that I would survive, and he had to be sure that he was truthful with them.

The darkest days followed the onset of the coma, when the disorder stubbornly refused to reveal itself. I became even less and less responsive and continued to sink deeper away. One evening, Bruce returned home and put on his happy face for the children so they wouldn't be frightened any more than they already were. After putting them to bed, he made a late phone call to the intensive care unit, probably knowing—and dreading—what he would hear, but feeling that he had to know nonetheless.

"This is Bruce Ford," he said. "I'm calling to see how my wife is doing. Is … is there any change?"

The nurse's guarded, but frank response was, "She's getting worse."

Medical Record, Beth Israel-Deaconess

May 24, 1998

5:06 AM Intensive Care, progress note:

Patient continues to respond only to pain or noxious stimuli [that is done to get a response from the patient, such as flinch. Examples include: rubbing on the sternum with knuckles or compressing at the base of the nail bed with a finger nail]. No movement of lower extremities or left upper extremity, all of which are stiff. Slight movement of right upper extremity, which is mostly flaccid … [Patient] continues with fevers. Lumbar puncture repeated, results pending. Tylenol given twice with fair effect.

—E. F. Paradise, RN

2:21 PM *Progress note:*

Patient's wedding and engagement rings and watch sent home with husband.

—J. A. Atterstrom, RN

Judy handed the rings to Bruce that afternoon as he prepared to return home. "Yes, I could see that you would want to get those off," Bruce told the nurse, who quietly made reference to the swelling caused by the intravenous needles.

I just tried to keep in mind the practical reason to take them off. I just wanted to maintain my composure, to avoid becoming emotional. I took them, quickly. I couldn't possibly have felt any lower. When I got home, I put them away, quickly, and went back to whatever I was doing, quickly. I had to keep my cool. I had to be able to go into a conference room and talk to six doctors, and I had to be able to go home and take care of two little kids.

—Bruce

Once the coma set in, it became apparent that the antiviral and antibacterial therapy that Dr. Zaleznik had started almost immediately upon my admission was not resulting in any progress. The emphasis shifted significantly to neurology. At this time, the doctors explained that they wanted to make some changes to make me "more comfortable." A patient can't be kept on an endotracheal tube, the temporary mechanism introduced to ensure that breathing continues without interruption, for an unlimited time. A tracheostomy would be required. For similar reasons, the doctors also would insert the PEG tube into my stomach for nutrition.

From these adjustments, my family understood the unspoken message. No one knew how long I would be in a coma or when, or if, I would emerge from it. The Beth Israel-Deaconess medical staff began to broach the subject of a long rehabilitation. A patient in what is known as a "persistent coma" no longer needed to be in an intensive care unit. Such a patient could be transferred to a rehabilitation hospital or elsewhere.

The scenarios playing out in the minds of my family and friends were not happy ones. Bruce, for one, began to wonder whether the medical people at Beth Israel-Deaconess felt they had done all that was possible.

Medical Record, Beth Israel-Deaconess

May 25, 1998

2:29 PM Intensive Care, progress note:

[Patient] remains intubated and ventilated with minimal secretions. All extremities are flaccid [with] no response. She will grimace with noxious stimuli ... Noted once to have very brief shoulder "vibrations" ... No obvious neurology change ... The plan is for a family meeting tomorrow afternoon. Have spoken with husband regarding impending discussions about trach, PEG, and rehab placement ... He seems to understand the reasoning for the trach and PEG; however, he is reluctant to discuss.

—R. M. Andwood, RN

3:34 PM Internal Medicine, progress note:

There continues to be little change in her neurology functions. Most likely etiology [cause] remains viral meningoencephalitis. Patient's husband is aware of likely need for extended rehab and probable trach/PEG and is in agreement.

—M. G. McLaughlin, MD

Radiology, final report:

As before, no abnormal foci of T2 hyperintensity are seen within the brain ... The head is tilted toward the left. The ventricles and cisterns appear remarkable ... Normal head MRI study with no abnormal enhancement following gadolinium [a dye used in MRI to help reveal certain pathologies given intravenously and has fewer side effects than the dye used in a CAT scan].

—(unsigned)

As the reports from radiology indicated, the MRIs again did not reveal any abnormality: normal upon normal results, eliciting no clues whatsoever. The doctors were stumped. The evil malady was playing its cards pretty close. There was no improvement. Although there were suspicions and theories about what had happened, there was no positive confirmation about the cause of the disorder and, therefore, no clear indication of what direction the treatment should take. It was a nasty, inexplicable situation—and one without hope.

Bruce finally decided it was time to call the Reverend Harold Babcock, our minister at the Unitarian Church in Newburyport. The days had begun, dangerously, to turn into weeks. Hope was slim to none, and he could put it off no longer. It was time to address the worst-case scenario.

"Harold," he began. "It's Bruce. Wendy is very sick. We don't know why; they don't know what it is. She's in a coma at Beth Israel. It doesn't look good at all."

"I am so sorry," Harold told him. "What would you like me to do?"

"I don't know. Just stand by, I guess. I don't know what's going to happen. It looks like she's probably going to die."

"I'll do anything you want me to do, Bruce. Here's my home phone number and my schedule. Marge knows how to reach me if I'm not in my office. I'll wait to hear from you."

Then I went to the beach. I had done everything I could think of to do. The kids were taken care of. There was nothing else for me to do, so I drove down to Plum Island. I found a stretch of sand where I could be alone. I prayed to the ocean.

It was the biggest thing I knew.

—Bruce

◆ ◆ ◆

One rainy evening, as Bruce and my mother drove home from Boston, he picked up a message from his mother. Mary Ford, who lived in Springfield, Massachusetts, desperately wanted to help. He returned the call as he approached the Tobin Bridge, high over Boston Harbor.

"Bruce," she announced vigorously, "there was an article in the paper out here today about a young woman who had an unusual neurological disorder that seems remarkably similar to Wendy's—and I know the family!"

Indeed, it was a propitious coincidence. Bruce listened intently as his mother related the specifics of the case. He anticipated that there would be dissimilarities that would make that case inapplicable, but he wanted to at least hear her out before moving on to try something else. He knew the reality, but he couldn't bear to lose hope—and he was thorough.

Like me, the young woman not only had experienced flu-like symptoms before she was stricken, but a direct cause to explain the neurological issue could not be identified. Like me, the young woman had suffered from a terrible headache. The other most dangerous parallel between the two cases was that, like mine, the doctors were unable to make a diagnosis or order treatment. Dr. Anthony Jackson, the neurologist in the Springfield case, admitted to flying by the seat of his pants in ultimately making his diagnosis. Like mine, the Springfield case was extremely rare and no clear solution presented itself.

Finally, in a desperate attempt to save the young woman's life, Dr. Jackson had administered steroids. The steroids worked by serving to reduce the inflammation around the young woman's cerebellum.

"Steroids" is the short way to refer to anabolic steroids, which, according to the *Encyclopedia of Drugs and Alcohol,* are the synthetic versions of the naturally occurring male sex hormone, testosterone. Because steroids suppress both inflammation and the immune system, it is unwise to administer them in an infectious situation because they could impede the body's own ability to fight the inflection.

One suspicion the doctors had was that my disorder was, in fact, infectious, and great care had to be taken in considering the use of steroids.

As Dr. Scammell later explained, "When somebody has a life-threatening disease, you want to give the body a chance to fight it off."

However, a high sedimentation rate was definitely present. In the words of Dr. David Trentham, the Beth Israel-Deaconess rheumatologist, the rate was "amazingly high." This indicated inflammation, particularly in the brain, rather than an infection as the underlying cause.

Mary Ford gave her son the telephone number of her family friend, and Bruce called her immediately.

> *The woman's mother had become something of an expert on her daughter's case and was able to share much valuable information. There were striking similarities between the two cases. I pulled the car over on the bridge during a torrential downpour. I had to be able to take down the information to share with the doctors the next day.*
>
> —Bruce

That dangerous phone call on the bridge marked the beginning of the awareness of the possibilities of steroids.

Back in Boston the next morning, Bruce was eager to meet with my doctors and share with them what he had learned the evening before. The doctors seemed surprised that Bruce knew of the potential that a steroid therapy might offer. Of course, they had considered steroids. They explained again that steroids could be useful in the case of inflammation; however, if the nature of the disease were infectious, steroids would have a serious negative effect.

But steroids were under consideration. The doctors simply needed confirmation that the cause was inflammation. They needed a clue.

◆ ◆ ◆

Meanwhile, the members of my family, as well as friends, were trying everything they could think of to reach me. Bruce placed a huge bouquet of Stargazer lilies at my bedside. These were the flowers he had courted me with the summer we met, twenty-two years earlier, on Martha's Vineyard. Their fragrance filled my room and spilled out into the corridor of the intensive care unit. He may have hoped that the strong scent of the lilies would somehow get through to me, and he knew that the nurses would enjoy them. He also brought in a beautiful photograph of our children and placed it at my bedside. He was trying to make sure that the doctors and nurses attending me would gain a sense of the life he hoped could be saved, and if I woke up—yes, *if*—he wanted the first thing I saw to be the picture of Westy and Lindsay.

Having adorned my bedside with such tenderness and consideration, and knowing there was nothing further he could do there, he resumed his role as general in the war. Bruce called all of my doctors, as well as all of our friends who were doctors. We had met Dr. Eliot Berson years before as neighbors in Boston's Back Bay. Bruce called Eliot, a renowned ophthalmologist at the Massachusetts Eye and Ear Infirmary and Harvard Medical School professor.

Bruce wanted to make sure that the best minds at Mass General would be in contact with the doctors at Beth Israel. Massachusetts General Hospital and Massachusetts Eye and Ear Infirmary are both Harvard Medical School teaching hospitals.

"You've got to get your team in touch with Morton Scwartz at Mass General," Eliot said. He immediately arranged for Dr. Scwartz, considered to be the dean of the study of infectious disease, to consult with my doctors at Beth Israel-Deaconess, many of whom had studied under him at Harvard Medical School.

"Another thing, Bruce," Eliot advised, "don't be afraid to get involved. I strongly urge you to play an active role: observe, monitor, and make suggestions. Don't hesitate. That advocacy is very important."

Bruce's personality was such that he needed little encouragement. However, the assurance coming from Eliot, and license that it was not only all right but the correct thing to do, carried great weight.

"Bruce was so sad," Mother later recalled. "We drove into Boston every day, and he was always on the phone, trying to find someone who had the knowledge to see you through this. I think that as soon as he felt he was making some progress along these lines, his spirits picked up. He was doing something, which made all of us feel better. He continually talked to the doctors about similar illnesses and the treatments that had brought those people back to health. The doctors, bless them, listened to all Bruce could tell them."

◆ ◆ ◆

I am certain that my persona as a wife and mother became more real as a result of Bruce's actions and advocacy, particularly in one area. It was Bruce who, with the doctors' blessings, arranged for my "coma sitters."

Eight years earlier, I had a different experience with a coma. When my father, Wendell Phillips Chapin, suffered a massive stroke in 1990 at the age of seventy-eight, he was rendered comatose. Over a period of several weeks, he intermittently failed, then stabilized. About halfway through this period, when it was thought he was about to die, the family was summoned. Bruce and I flew in from Boston. My sister flew in from Vancouver. My brothers came in from London and northern Michigan. We gathered and waited while trying to comfort Mom, who was, of course, holding up remarkably well. Dad ultimately stabilized during this time, and because we didn't know how much longer he might remain in that condition, the family made the decision to disperse.

Before Bruce and I made our return to Boston, we went to the hospital one last time. Dad's nurse gently suggested that I go into his room to say goodbye. She pulled the door shut so that Dad and I could have privacy. I was not prepared for that time alone with him. I had not anticipated that unwritten tradition that nurses would surely know about—the last goodbye.

It was ironic. I was literally full of life, seven months pregnant with my first child, a son who would be his grandfather's namesake. Being face-to-face with my father for what I understood would be the last time, I wondered whether I could reach him in his physical prison. Would he know I was there? Would he recognize my voice? What do I say? I had nothing planned. I clasped his hand and began talking. I tried to recount the reasons he had been such a great father.

"Dad," I said, "I have learned so much from you in so many ways. You are so very, very good and beloved by everyone who has ever known you." I told him why I had turned out the way I had (all the positives, at least) because of him.

"I love you so much," I told him through my tears. "You will always be with me in my heart." I looked at him and wondered what he heard, what he knew. *Am I getting through to him?* Then, slowly, he began to move. I was transfixed. *What is happening?* At that moment, he shifted his upper body and slowly, laboriously turned his head to face me where I stood.

"Dad, can you hear me?" I asked, amazed. "You *can* hear me, can't you?"

I swooped down on him, kissed his forehead, and caressed his cheek. I never forgot that moment and came to realize, much later, how excruciating and arduous it must have been for him to move his body and turn his head to me in that way. I always believed that this single, superhuman effort was his signal that he *was* able to hear me and that I *did* get through to him.

It was the last thing he ever did for me in his lifetime.

◆ ◆ ◆

Judy Atterstrom, my primary nurse, saw everyone who came into intensive care and made sure they had been approved by Bruce. My great friend Cathy

Ebling and Mother have both said I actually looked beautiful, which seemed hard to believe. Mothers do love to observe their children sleeping, but perhaps I was just finally quiet, for once!

"I remembered you as a baby," Mom had told me, "being sent to Wendell and me when we thought perhaps we would not have any more children." I was the fourth of four, six years after their third child. "I remembered watching you sleep in your bassinet between our beds and thinking what a precious bundle we have here. You seemed to be no trouble at all."

All of a sudden, however, I was a lot of trouble, and I was certainly asleep, big time. Visitors said I looked like myself, despite the medical paraphernalia. According to one visitor, "that great hair," which in reality is a head full of thick, stubborn cowlicks, "seemed always in place." However, what struck those with the courage, and the clearance, to visit me in the early intensive care days more than anything was the stillness. Foster would tell me later that I looked absolutely dead.

As Judy put it, despite what Cathy and Mom charitably thought, I was not at my best. She was certain I didn't want the world beating a path to my door. But with the hope that such familiar voices might perhaps awaken something in me, Bruce consulted with the doctors about having a few of my nearest and dearest come to the intensive care unit to sit and talk to me. These people were my "coma sitters," the most magnificent of friends and family: Cathy and her husband, Hilly; Foster, and Tim Hollingworth from John Hancock; my mother; and Bruce's sister and sister-in-law. I could only imagine what they must have gone through. I have no memory of that time, but I later understood that it was an ordeal for each of them.

Terri Ford, Bruce's sister-in-law, drove up from Cape Cod numerous times to sit with me. One day she brought a music box that played "Ebb Tide," which Judy wound up again and again before placing it on my pillow. Bruce's sister, Nancy, drove up from Croton-on-Hudson, New York, to be with me and help out at home, and she often brought her daughter, Olivia, to cheer up her cousins.

> *Dear Nancy, she just took over. She took care of the children, planned the dinner, did the laundry, and even cut the grass. All this allowed me to be able to drive into Boston with Bruce and talk to you and hold your hand more than I would have been able to do otherwise.*
>
> —Billie Chapin

Hilly and Cathy Ebling could barely speak about those days and weeks in the intensive care unit.

> *I just sat down and reminisced about all our great times together. I brought up the wonderful memories of being up at Tilden Pond* [our old camp in Maine], *being out on the water, and all our wild weekends living it up in Boston and New York—and points in between.*
>
> —Cathy Ebling

She recalled our years of limousines and swishy parties when we lived in the city. We went through those years with some style and spunk. We had a charmed life and spent years with dear and fun-loving people before the arrival of beautiful children. How quickly life had changed: from sailing Penobscot Bay and dancing in Newport to being a mother who was barely alive in the intensive care unit of Beth Israel-Deaconess Medical Center. What a disparity of worlds.

Cathy would run into people during the time I was hospitalized. They would greet her with the usual, "Hi, how are you?"

"Fine, thanks," she would say, while thinking all the while, "*Well, actually not very well. You see, my best friend seems to be dying, and nobody knows what to do for her.*"

Hilly Ebling felt similarly. "It wasn't easy," he would tell me later. "None of us had ever gone through anything like that. I remember leaving the bank to go to that place, knowing why I was going, what was happening—knowing the uncertainty."

> *I tracked my journey: Leaving State Street. Driving through Boston, through Back Bay. It was our old neighborhood, where we met all those years ago. Such fun ... Down to Beth Israel-Deaconess Medical Center: East Campus, Main Entrance. Going up in the elevator. What am I going to see? Ninth Floor, Medical Intensive Care Unit. Room Number One.*
>
> *You were so still. When I got there, I just went into a monologue, talked about our times together, the old camp ... It was strange. I knew you couldn't talk, but I wondered if you could hear me, could understand, somehow, from wherever you were.*
>
> —Hilly Ebling

Tim Hollingworth and I had been colleagues for more than a decade at John Hancock. Coworkers had described us as an old married couple. We bantered; we bickered; we understood each other; and we had a great time. The year before I moved my office from the twenty-seventh floor to the fifty-fourth floor and a new department. No more than two months later, Tim's new position landed him in the office next door to mine. We were delighted by the turn of events, the coincidence. He was the best of pals, a tender and courageous soul, as events would bear out.

Colleagues were so worried about Tim during that frightening time. "He was pale. He never smiled," Terri Nuti, our department secretary, later related. "I would go to his office several times a day, just to check on him and make sure he was all right."

Another colleague recalled, "The fifty-fourth floor was so quiet during that time, it was like a morgue. People huddled in little groups, whispering. We heard words like 'coma' and 'can't believe it.' No one laughed. No one smiled."

Foster didn't make it in to my room on the first try.

"When Foster first came," Judy would relate, "I didn't know who he was. He said you worked for him, and I just wanted to make sure that people who came to be with you had been cleared by the family. Then, of course, Bruce said it would be good to have him there because he was a friend whose familiar voice might be a comfort.

"Once he got here, it was so obvious to me that here was a person who really admired, and loved, my patient."

It required extraordinary courage and selflessness for Foster to come to the hospital. Twelve years earlier, almost to the month and in the same ward, his wife, the beloved Julika, lost her battle with cancer.

> *I will never forget walking down that hall, seeing my great friend in that place hooked up to all the intensive care equipment—all the tubes, lines, wires, all the electrical monitors, the catheter. It was pretty daunting. I just took a couple of deep breaths.*
>
> *It felt like a wake.*
>
> —Foster Aborn

But he and the rest of my coma sitters found their courage. I am convinced that their presence helped me; they all provided a mysterious world of good.

Bruce found it difficult to spend time sitting with me. He had a strong sliver of hope, but he also knew that there was a good chance that I was going to die, and it was difficult for him to see me hooked up to all the lines, tubes, and the rest of the ICU paraphernalia. His way of handling the crisis was to work at something. He was doing all he could to help save me; he was on his mission and felt that his time would be better spent elsewhere, working.

Indeed, he was afraid I was checking out, and he felt he had to pace himself. No one had any idea how long I'd be in that condition.

Judy Atterstrom made an interesting observation. She said she could tell that I was determined.

"Even in the coma?" I asked her months later. "How do you tell if someone in a coma is determined?"

"You can just *tell*," she said. "There's just something *there*, an inner strength that can be sensed."

Judy couldn't know me because, in a very real sense I was absent. However, she said she came to understand me and gain a sense of the person I was from the people who surrounded me. She supposed I was much like my tribe.

"The devotion of the people surrounding you was really something to see," she told me. "They were so dynamic, supportive, and strong. They seemed to have a willingness to do whatever they could to bring you back."

♦ ♦ ♦

Meanwhile, Dr. Scammell continued with his research and also consulted with numerous other neurologists throughout the Boston medical network, regardless of their hospital affiliation. He contacted people nationwide whose experience or expertise might help him solve the riddle of the mysterious affliction that had so suddenly felled an otherwise healthy and strong young woman. What would bring her out of the coma? What would bring her back?

After one week, the common wisdom seemed to point to encephalitis as the cause, which was often fatal. But Dr. Scammell would not be satisfied with that diagnosis.

"I just couldn't accept that this young woman kept getting sicker and sicker and that nothing more could be done," he would later tell me.

Early on, he suspected the problem to be acute disseminating [or demyelinating] encephalomyelitis (ADEM), but he needed confirmation in order to proceed. Indeed, he could not proceed without confirmation. He was searching for a clue, an indication of some sort, any sort, to support his hypothesis. The evidence pointed heavily to an infection, primarily because the brain MRIs continued to register normal. It was unlikely that there was an inflammation of the white matter, which would indicate ADEM. Other factors that pointed to infection were the consistently high fevers and high white blood cell count. With such evidence, viral encephalitis seemed to be the much more likely diagnosis.

Again, without a positive diagnosis, there could be no treatment.

Medical Record, Beth Israel-Deaconess

May 26, 1998

5:20 AM Intensive Care, progress note:

No significant change on neurology status. She is deeply comatose, responding intermittently to painful or noxious stimuli. At other times, she is completely unresponsive. Not observed to move extremities. Does turn head and make chewing motions ... Temperature down with Tylenol and cooling blanket ... Patient repositioned, [foot] splints on and off as recommended by occupational therapist.

Anticipate family meeting today to discuss trach, PEG, rehab placement. [We] need to have our team—infectious diseases, neurology, social services, nursing—as well as family present.

—E. F. Paradise, RN

1:16 PM Intensive Care, progress note:

EEG [electroencephalogram] today with suggestion of seizure activity. [Patient] begun on Dilantin.

Assessment and plan: Encephalitis, etiology unclear, infectious (viral) most probable. Steroids have not been recommended by infectious diseases and neurology services because of lack of etiology and evidence. However, duration of fevers and high sedimentation rates [a nonspecific reference indicating inflammation or infection] ... [and] months of nonspecific "fatigue" suggests some possible underlying rheumatic disorder ... Neurological exam is difficult at this point and EEG suggests seizures. Family meeting today to discuss poor prognosis for rapid recovery even should she stabilize and her neurological status improve.

—H. Yu, MD

For Bruce, this was the most hellish time. In addition to the persistent medical mystery, the inability of the doctors to make a diagnosis, and the frustration and despair at the consequent lack of treatment, I was experiencing a swiftly accelerating deterioration.

At this time, the doctors began to explore another therapy that they hoped might end the coma: plasmapheresis. This is a blood filtration process that rids the plasma—the liquid in which the different kinds of blood cells are suspended—of harmful antibodies. It had been applied in similar cases, but the doctors were unsure how it would affect the outcome of my case. If I did have viral encephalitis, plasmapheresis might make my condition worse—just as a program of steroids would.

Medical Record, Beth Israel-Deaconess

May 26, 1998

Infectious Diseases Attending: Clinically unchanged. Gagging on tube; otherwise unresponsive ... We thought about HIV [human immunodeficiency virus] only to consider any complicating infection that might pertain, not because we thought HIV was causing her illness ... Likely worth getting an opinion from risk management on proxy HIV testing, for future reference.

—D. Zaleznik

Infectious Diseases:

No major events overnight. Still comatose. Family visiting much of the day. Need impeccable care to avoid superinfection. Team concerned regarding the legalities of proxy consent for HIV test ... Would doubt she is HIV-positive.

—[ID]

With only a few dozen ADEM cases on record, there was scant material to reference, and what material there was shed little light. For the neurologists at Beth Israel-Deaconess, it was like starting from scratch. But led by Dr. Scammell, they rallied to the challenge. Despite the frustrations and unending mystery, he pushed the team to persevere.

He made numerous calls to people who had written about ADEM. He consulted with a number of other doctors who collectively represented tremendous experience in clinical neurology. One in particular was Dr. Dan Kanter, formerly of Brigham and Women's Hospital (BWH), which was another of the Harvard Medical School teaching hospitals in Boston. Dr. Kanter had written papers on the treatment of ADEM that Dr. Scammell found particularly helpful.

I had no hesitation to call for advice at BWH. Even though the parent organizations of Beth Israel-Deaconess and Brigham and Women's were economic competitors, there were good lines of medical communication in Boston. When confronted with a clinical problem that is particularly challenging, I, and most other MDs I know, will first discuss the mystery among their local network of advisors and then search the medical literature to find the best national help.

—T. Scammell, MD

Dr. Scammell explained that the spinal taps and the clinical course of the disorder suggested ADEM, but the brain MRIs kept coming back normal. This continued to confound them all. Lou Kaplan, one of the world's experts in stroke and perhaps the most renowned neurologist in Boston, told Dr. Scammell it sounded like encephalitis.

Yet Dr. Scammell never gave up. He kept sending me for the MRIs, hoping against hope that they would somehow give him the clue he needed. But it wasn't promising. In the few documented cases of ADEM, the indications of the disorder were apparent from the earliest MRIs, and ADEM didn't usually result in coma. Within a very rare category, my case appeared to be singularly rare.

Medical Record, Beth Israel-Deaconess

May 26, 1998

Neurology Consultant Attending:

Patient now comatose on ventilator. No eye opening to voice or nail bed pressure. EEG: Rhythmic slow activity with suggestion of ongoing seizures.

Impression: Coma is secondary to encephalitis. Continues to decline clinically, as EEG now suggests subclinical seizures. [Most seizures are obvious, jerking of the limbs or a sudden change in behavior. Subclinical seizures affect only a small part of the brain and may affect brain function so subtly that the change cannot be noticed by the observer. Alternatively, a person can be so sick— paralyzed or comatose—that the seizures are obscured by the other findings.] Nonconvulsive status epileptics usually can be recognized by ... eye movements such as lid fluttering, so I do not think she is actually in status [of having epileptic seizures]. Still, she is at risk for developing seizures, and treatment with Dilantin ... should be helpful. Aim for level of 10–20 unless overt seizures develop in which case higher dose may be recommended.

—T. Scammell, MD

One afternoon, a young foreign resident motioned to Bruce to follow him out into the hall. His spirits sank. As it had been on so many previous occasions, Bruce's first thought was, *This is it. He's going to tell me she has a half hour.*

"Many things we have tested," the young doctor told him, "but there is one test we have not done."

He was referring to the test for HIV, an alarmingly real possibility because of my birthing history. I had required massive transfusions for postpartum hemorrhaging when Westy was born, back in 1990.

Other doctors soon brought the issue out into the open. Mother remembers seeing one doctor call Bruce aside, then look at her over his shoulder. "I found out later that he was asking Bruce's permission to run an HIV test, about the only test they hadn't run."

However, this presented an ethical dilemma. By law, in order for someone to be tested for the AIDS virus, consent must be given by the individual to be tested. Bruce and Mother were adamant that I would agree to be tested, if only I could speak or nod my head to show that I understood. They were right. I definitely would have agreed to the test. Not fully aware of the potential legal ramifications, Bruce pleaded with the doctors: "Test her *today*—please."

He was met by silence as the doctors wrestled with their quandary. Lawsuits had been brought against hospitals when HIV testing occurred without the consent of the individual in question. The unfortunate facts of the matter:

1. The patient had a potentially fatal affliction, the cause of which was still a mystery, and treatment was impossible without the risk of further injury or death.
2. The patient had a major blood transfusion in 1990.
3. It could take eight years or more for the symptoms of AIDS to surface, and her son was approaching his eighth birthday.
4. The patient could not speak to indicate her consent for the testing.
5. If the test could shed light on the affliction and lead to a diagnosis and treatment, the patient's family strongly desired testing.

The hospital was between the twin perils, Scylla and Charybdis.

That night, Bruce spoke with Dr. McLaughlin, the head of the intensive care unit, and renewed his pleas.

"I am sorry, Bruce," Dr. McLaughlin reaffirmed. "Our hands are tied. By law, we cannot test for HIV without the patient's consent."

Medical Record, Beth Israel-Deaconess

May 26, 1998

Intensive Care Attending: Family meeting from 4:30–5:00 PM in conference room with primary nurse, intern, social worker, myself, and patient's husband and mother. Two main issues were discussed. [One was the] possible utility of checking HIV status. Patient's husband and mother adamant about fact that she would agree to testing if we felt this would provide valuable information that might alter our current course. They also have requested a second opinion from infectious disease services, which we will be happy to arrange. It is not clear that HIV testing at this point will change what we are doing [but] will provide with testing if infectious diseases consultants feel strongly that this would be helpful. Also discussed that patient is facing a prolonged course requiring intubation. Family has agreed to tracheostomy and PEG.

—R. Wright, MD

My condition continued to worsen. My breathing had become more labored, and my ability to breathe on my own was now a major concern. The discussion of the tracheostomy, in addition to the concern with HIV, was the nadir, for Bruce.

Not only is Wendy comatose, Bruce thought, *but she's having trouble breathing on her own, and now there's the possibility of AIDS looming before us.*

The tracheostomy, or trach, had been under discussion for several days. A trach is a surgical incision in the neck, of the trachea, for the purpose of making an artificial breathing hole. A tube also was necessary, as a protective measure, to ensure that a patient's breathing continued uninterrupted. The staff explained this carefully to Mom and Bruce over the course of several days, to help prepare them for the reality of it.

♦ ♦ ♦

Dr. Scammell and others repeatedly noted in the medical record that there was no response to nail bed pressure, the litmus test of awareness. It was as deep a coma as possible: death's door.

"We squeeze people's nail beds to see if they respond to pain," Judy would later tell me. "It's very painful. I usually don't do this, however, as there are enough neurologists and MDs around to do it. As a nurse, I cause pain my own way just doing my normal thing."

Among the dozens of medical experts who worked for days to determine what was wrong were the rheumatologists. They were brought in for their knowledge about the body's immune system. Although they, too, considered ADEM, they also felt it prudent to hold off on steroids. Their concern was vasculitis, an inflammation of the blood vessels through an autoimmune process that could lead to strokes, seizures, and secondary inflammation of the central nervous system. By the time the rheumatologists, headed by Dr. Trentham, were called in, I was on a respirator. He echoed what others had said.

> *We're often called in to try to unravel an inexplicable case. Yet, within this universe of highly unusual cases, this one stood out as a diagnostic dilemma of the first order. The situation was so very confounding because of the rapidity with which the coma came on. Nothing seemed to fit. Nothing meshed with reality. It seemed like we were trying to take a round peg and fit it into a square hole.*
>
> —D. Trentham, MD

Rheumatology conducted a magnetic resonance angio scan (MRA) that employed specific ways to look at blood vessels. The rheumatologists looked for evidence of pleocytosis—inflammatory white blood cells in the cerebral spinal fluid. They also conducted an antinuclear antibody (ANA) test for lupus, another autoimmune disease that could attack a variety of organs, including the brain.

On the subject of steroids, Dr. Trentham had begun to think that because my situation was so grave, neither steroids nor plasmapheresis would be detrimental. I was in such bad shape that without intervention of some sort it seemed just a matter of time before I would die.

On May 26, Bruce asked for a meeting with all the doctors. It took place in a conference room on the ninth floor of intensive care, just steps from my room. Bruce made what he called his final Knute Rockne speech. At this point, he was feeling about as low as he possibly could, but he was trying anything to keep the doctors going, to keep them from giving up, as hopeless as it seemed.

"Thank you for coming," he began. "I know how busy you are. I just wanted to let you know how much we appreciate all of your incredible work. I thought it was important for you to know how we feel. I know that it seems hopeless, but I hope you keep trying. I want to encourage that. Please keep trying, as impossible as it must seem. She is so special."

The frustration factor among the hospital staff was tremendous.

We care about every patient who comes through here, but when the situation centers on someone our own age—the age of most of the doctors and nurses—and someone, again like many of us, with young children, it makes it very easy to identify. We all thought, there but for the grace of God ...

—T. Scammell, MD

Superimposed on the ingratiating aspects of the case was the enigma, the mystery of it all: What in the world is going on? We thought life is very unjust. It seemed like an act of the devil.

—D. Trentham, MD

With such a terrifying case, it is often difficult to be objective. Sometimes there is a tendency to overdo, to work so urgently that too much therapy is offered. It becomes a race against time and, perhaps, fate.

When someone is that sick, we feel a tremendous sense of urgency. The alternative really galvanizes everyone.

—T. Scammell, MD

The alternative, of course, being death.

◆ ◆ ◆

Medical Record, Beth Israel-Deaconess

May 27, 1998

5:26 AM Intensive Care, progress note:

Remains unresponsive, no spontaneous movements noted. Does not open eyes, occasionally moans and shakes head when doing mouth care. Biting down on tongue ... Occasionally having left-sided chill-like tremors that respond well to intravenous Ativan; remains on Dilantin ... Remains unresponsive. Neurology status worsening.

—P. A. Chabre, RN

♦ ♦ ♦

One afternoon during this time, when Bruce and Mother returned home, they cheered themselves up for the children. They also attempted to catch up with the minutiae of daily family life. Bruce had picked up the mail, and out popped a note from Joanie Purinton, whom we fondly referred to as the Queen of Charity on the North Shore. Inside the note was a photograph her husband, Dick, had taken of B.G. and me on May 2nd. It was the evening of a benefit dinner-dance at the historic Lowell's Boat Shop, less than two weeks before I fell ill. In the photograph, Bruce and I shared dessert as we watched the auction activity. Joanie wrote:

Dear Bruce & Wendy,

Thank you for joining us & always supporting the good causes.

Wendy looks chic from every angle, as always.

Have a happy spring,

Love,

Joanie P.

The note was dated May 19, 1998. Joanie had written it on the day of my admission to Beth Israel-Deaconess. By the time Bruce received it, with the photograph of our last festive occasion, I had already slipped into the abyss. It was a dramatic contrast to the current reality.

♦ ♦ ♦

Medical Record, Beth Israel-Deaconess

May 27, 1998

6:57 PM Intensive Care, progress note:

Essentially unchanged. Minimally responsive ... Periods of apnea intermittently ... Husband spoke with infectious diseases, neurology, and intensive care teams as well as social services today. He continues to search for answers. Patient's mother also in. [They] appear very supportive of each other.

—J. A. Atterstrom, RN

Neurology Consultant Attending:

Please try to keep fevers down, as hyperthermia may aggravate ... injury.

—T. Scammell, MD

Social Work:

As notes reflect, family/team meeting yesterday where team outlined course of events to date and answered questions of patient's husband and mother. Patient's family asking appropriate questions of team, understandably quite concerned regarding patient's medical status and quite able to articulate their fears and concerns. Patient's family also able to speak with social workers regarding age-related issues as to how and what to explain to patient's children, three and eight years old. Patient's husband interested in finding outside consultation "down the line" as he feels that this may be needed at greater length ... Team has also addressed patient's eventual need for rehab with family, but patient's husband feels adamant that patient not be moved until the cause of patient's condition is known.

—L. Cahey, Lic. SW

Dangerously, the days had turned into weeks. Despite the suspicion of ADEM, the pivotal tests, the MRIs, continued to come back normal.

"The collective depression of the house staff and the nursing staff, up there in the intensive care unit, was profound," Dr. Trentham later recalled. "The question was: what mutant virus is destroying this person?"

Medical Record, Beth Israel-Deaconess

May 28, 1998

6:28 AM Intensive Care, progress note:

No changes noted; remains unresponsive. Does shake head occasionally with painful stimuli ... Does not open eyes to voice or to stimuli.

—(unsigned)

2:06 PM Internal Medicine, progress note:

Remains febrile, although fever curve and WBC (white blood count) declining ... 1 kilogram weight gain over 24 hours, still below admission weight ... Trach today for expected long-term requirement for airway protection ... PEG placed for long-term feedings. Will initiate when cleared by surgery.

—M. McLaughlin, MD

Infectious Diseases Attending:

Patient got trach and PEG today. [Patient is] lying flat, gagging a bit, but breathing. May have [had] some subtle facial movements today.

—D. Zaleznik, MD

The medical people don't like to keep the endotracheal tube in place more than two weeks because it may cause erosion of the trachea. The tracheostomy performed on May 28, one week and two days after my admission to Beth Israel-Deaconess, was the standard practice for patients who, it was felt, would have to be vented for longer than a fortnight.

"We knew it would be a long time, if ever, before you would be able to breathe on your own," Judy would later explain.

The breathing apparatus, with its fluttery rubber membrane plugged into my neck, had a chilling effect on visitors.

It was so mechanical and ... contrived ... so clinical. It was awful, knowing that they had to cut into you to put it in. My God, *I thought, how does this thing work?*

—Foster Aborn

The situation was so grave, and getting worse. The general feeling was that you wouldn't pull out of it anytime soon.

—D. Trentham, MD

Meanwhile, there were signs of medical disagreement.

Medical Record, Beth Israel-Deaconess

May 28, 1998

Neurology Consultant Attending:

I understand that plasmapheresis has been raised as a possible therapy. If there were evidence for an autoimmune process (such as acute disseminated encephalomyelitis, etc.), plasmapheresis might be of some benefit. However, any autoimmune process that produced such widespread CNS [central nervous system] dysfunction should have raised T2 on her MRI. Additionally, plasmapheresis might remove beneficial antibodies that she has generated to combat her encephalitis. Thus, I feel plasmapheresis is unlikely to be beneficial, and could possibly be harmful. If you think it would be helpful, I'd be happy to meet with the intensive care/infectious diseases/rheumatology teams to discuss her case.

—T. Scammell, MD

◆ ◆ ◆

Judy approached Bruce one afternoon on another devastating question. "Does Wendy have a living will?" she asked.

Bruce and I did have such documents. We had signed them in the fall of 1994, in the office of our attorney, Bill O'Flaherty, blithely thinking we were merely preparing to make things easy for our children, decades down the road. Westy was then four. I was three months pregnant with Lindsay.

"We should probably have it on hand," said Judy, quietly.

Now, on a beautiful spring morning, Bruce waited in his attorney's office on the North Shore, while down in Boston, his wife lay dying. Many people, of course, have had experience with living wills, but usually in conjunction with the care of aged, failing parents. But who could imagine what must have gone on in Bruce's mind during this errand to retrieve a document signed just a few years earlier as their young son cavorted on the floor of Bill's conference room? A piece of paper with a signature, *her* signature, that could pave the way for an order to remove her life-support systems, the life-support systems of the mother of a three-year-old daughter and a seven-year-old son—*her treasures*. How to tell the children? How to *be*, afterward? How to go on as a single parent—a widower?

Who knows what goes on in the mind of a person at such a time?

A living will.

Its legalistic language took on a sudden gravitas that we had not come close to appreciating at the signing less than four years earlier:

Living Will Declaration and Health Care Proxy

I. Living Will Declaration.

To my family, physicians, and to all hospitals, health care facilities and health care providers in whose care I may be hereafter, and to any individual who may become responsible for my health or welfare, and to any court having jurisdiction over my person or property.

I, WENDY CHAPIN FORD, being of sound mind, willfully and voluntarily make known my desires that my dying shall not be artificially prolonged under the circumstances set forth below, and do declare:

If at any time, I should have an incurable injury, disease, or illness certified to be a terminal condition by two (2) physicians who have personally examined me, one of whom shall be my attending physician, and the physicians have determined that my death will occur whether or not life-sustaining procedures are utilized and where the application of life-sustaining procedures would serve only to artificially prolong the dying process, I direct that such procedures be withheld or withdrawn, and that I be permitted to die naturally with only the administration of medication or the performance of any medical procedure deemed necessary to provide me with comfort, care or to alleviate pain.

To the extent that artificial and so-called "heroic" measures are required to keep me alive, I request that I be allowed to die a dignified death, that I not be kept alive by such measures, that medication be liberally and mercifully administered to me to alleviate suffering even though this may hasten the moment of my death, and that any action be taken or withheld, as the case may be, so as not to unreasonably prolong my death, nor destroy the dignity of my life.

I hereby release and discharge all doctors, surgeons, lawyers, hospitals, health care agencies, all members of my family and all friends and other persons acting for me or on my behalf under the provisions of this Declaration, so that it is clear that all are free from any legal liability …

I hereby appoint the following person as my health care agent to have authority to make health care decisions on my behalf if it is determined pursuant to Section 6 of Chapter 201D, [Massachusetts General Laws], that I lack the capacity to make or to communicate health care decisions:

Name: BRUCE GRAHAM FORD

If BRUCE GRAHAM FORD is not available, willing, or competent to serve and is not expected to become available, willing, or competent to make a timely decision given my medical circumstances; or if he is disqualified from acting on my behalf pursuant to other requirements of Chapter 201D, then I appoint the following person to act as my alternate health care agent to make health care decisions on my behalf:

Name: S. KIM CHAPIN

Signed: WENDY CHAPIN FORD

Date: October 6, 1994

It certainly fit all the definitions of torture. Torture takes place over time. You are made to feel helpless, and that any possible effort is futile, and that there is no light at the end of the tunnel. You're pushed to your limits, but you're not told the limits. It was torture, exactly.

At the same time, it was all streamlined. Judy asked for it, I put it on the list of things to do, and I gave it to her the next day. But I didn't spend a lot of time thinking about it.

It wasn't part of my plan to have to use it.

—Bruce

♦ ♦ ♦

During these darkest of times, Bruce received a phone call that would stand out among the countless others that were coming in from friends and relatives around the country. This call was from John Constable in Hershey, Pennsylvania. John was a dear, older friend of ours and the father of my sister-in-law, Anne Constable. Bruce was unaware of it at the time, but John was suffering from heart disease and would himself die before the year was out.

"I just wanted to say how concerned Anne [his wife] and I have been about the situation with Wendy up in Boston," John said. "We've been remembering all those great times we shared together at your old camp in Maine.

"Tilden Pond was such a special place, wasn't it? Do you remember the day young Anne took Nicky, who must have been about three at the time, out on the pond to fish? I still have a great photograph of the two of them in your old red canoe, showing off a big bass they'd caught. Big smiles all around …"

What John said next had a particular resonance for Bruce.

"I remember talking to Nick and his older brother Alex about what to do with the catch," John continued. "Coincidentally, I had just read an article about how to release a fish, and the boys agreed that it should go back into the pond. So, we massaged the fish—lifted its gills to get them going again—

then slipped the fish gently back into the water. And isn't it amazing how they just take right off and go when they're put back?"

It was amazing. And for Bruce, and so many others, that is exactly what they hoped would happen with me—that at some point I would return to my element and just take off and go.

♦ ♦ ♦

On the morning of Friday, May 29, Bruce walked into my room and found Dr. McLaughlin sitting in a chair by the window. I, as usual, lay motionless in my bed, the sounds of my labored, mechanically assisted breathing, with its ominous rhythm punctuating the quiet of the intensive care unit.

"We have found some small lesions on the white matter of the brain," Dr. McLaughlin quietly announced.

Bruce was stunned. *How much more can I take?* he thought.

"It's actually good news," the doctor quickly explained. "It could be the breakthrough, the clue we've been seeking. Now we can initiate a treatment."

Bruce could hardly believe it, after all he had been through. He was hopeful, but guardedly so.

The operative event actually had occurred late the previous afternoon.

Medical Record, Beth Israel-Deaconess

May 28, 1998

4:33 PM Radiology, findings:

The brain parenchymal white matter is diffusely abnormal in appearance with patchy, poor marginated areas of T2 signal hyperintensity which involve both cerebral hemispheres ... Impressions: Diffusely abnormal brain scan with appearances most suggestive of an acute demyelinating process or diffuse encephalitis.

—M. Silvera, MD
—M. Patel, MD

... the intensity of white matter disease, the fact that this illness followed a mild viral URI [upper respiratory infection] and her relatively normal peripheral white count are supportive of ADEM.

—T. Scammell, MD

At last! The lesions that pointed to ADEM finally revealed themselves in this MRI that produced the first abnormal results, enabling the doctors—liberating them—to initiate a treatment. They would treat this as an inflammation process. It was agreed that steroids were the safest first course. If that did not produce results, then the next step would be plasmapheresis, the complicated blood filtration process considered earlier.

"Why the lesions were not apparent on the early MRI scans is a fascinating question," Dr. Scammell told me some months afterward. "Clearly, your brain and spinal cord were malfunctioning early in your illness, but MRI scans, though amazing, are not perfect.

"MRI scans are good at detecting brain edema, the swelling that accompanies inflammation. Although your neurons were misbehaving, there may not have been enough edema early on for the MRI to detect. Usually in ADEM, the edema is very obvious."

This is why the early MRIs kept registering normal results. This compounded the mystery and dangerously hampered the diagnosis and search for treatment.

"Although bugs and ticks can cause neurological disease, ADEM is most likely explained as a very abnormal response within the immune system," Dr. Scammell went on to explain. "A normal response of the immune system is to attack bacteria or viruses that cause harm to an individual. An abnormal response, such as ADEM, is that in which the immune cells attack the wrong thing: in this case, your myelin. Your system produced antibodies that, by some unfortunate coincidence, were not as selective as they should have been and attacked your central nervous system. This was a brain and spinal cord disorder."

This pivotal discovery cleared the way for megadose steroid therapy that began early in the afternoon on May 29. Dr. Scammell initiated a therapy consisting of 1,000 milligrams of Solumedrol, a high-pulse steroid. The steroid was administered intravenously for each of the next five days.

The therapy began with hope, but there was no guarantee that it would work.

Medical Record, Beth Israel-Deaconess

May 29, 1998

6:47 AM Intensive Care, progress note:

No neuro changes. No spontaneous movements noted, other than facial grimaces with pain.

—P.A. Chabre, RN

12:36 PM Intensive Care, progress note:

Patient has had many more facial grimaces today. When asked to open her eyes, she is able to lift her eyebrows, but the eyes don't open. She winces when limbs are stimulated and tape is removed from skin.

—J. Crivell, RN

1:06 PM Intensive Care, progress note:

MRI/MRA/MRV ... of head and spine reveal demyelination on preliminary reading ... With evidence of demyelination ... [and] after consultation with neurology and infectious diseases, will initiate a trial of high-dose steroids, continue Dilantin, check EEG. PEG placed yesterday. Will start tube feeds today and advance as tolerated.

—H. Yu, MD

10:43 PM Intensive Care, progress note:

No change from earlier notes documenting her status today ... Patient's husband states, "This has been a pretty good bad day," meaning that at least there is a working diagnosis and intervention with the steroids ... [He] feels well supported by the institution.

—C. J. Perella, RN

Chapter Three

The Awakening

May 30 was a remarkable day. It was the occasion of the first positive development that anyone dared note during the entire episode thus far. Dr. Scammell's overview, as well as the progress notes for the day, showed some actual progress, for the first time.

Medical Notes, Beth Israel-Deaconess

May 30, 1998

Neurology Consultant Attending:

Small but remarkable improvement overnight! She now occasionally opens her eyes to voice, possibly followed midline commands ("open/close your eyes"), briefly fixed and followed my face. Now has very brisk facial grimace to pain in nail beds and severe left facial weakness is evident. Her definite improvement agrees strongly that she must have ADEM. Considering her steady downhill course in the last week, I find it unlikely that a viral encephalitis should improve so rapidly. As long as she continues to improve, would continue five-day course of Solumedrol.

—T. Scammell, MD

5:31 AM Intensive Care, progress note:

Although upper and lower extremity weakness continues without change, patient is able to grimace, yawn, and is coughing when stimulated during suctioning ...

—F. E. Arlia, RN

12:33 PM Intensive Care, progress note:

Some mild improvement in neuro status with increased responsiveness to noxious stimuli.

—W. Stead, MD

6:17 PM Intensive Care, progress note:

Patient's eyelids flicker, appears to attempt to open eyes upon request but unable to do so. Yawning, grimacing with discomfort when turning, etc. No movement from upper or lower extremities.

—E. M. Condon, RN

The overnight clinical improvement completely vindicated the MRI findings that revealed the lesions, as well as the subsequent, conclusive diagnosis and the decision to administer steroids. With the beginning of the treatment, I began to regain consciousness.

"The effects of the steroid therapy marked the beginning of a slow return to awareness," Dr. Scammell explained to me later. "As one learns to read the signposts of infant development, it can be understood that the little baby things began to come back first. Like an infant, you initially began to fix and follow faces. In time, you would sit and swallow."

For a person who had lost so much, the little things were significant. It wasn't at all apparent what functions I ultimately would be able to recover. No one could tell how far I might go.

But I was alive.

At first, you opened your eyes but then shut them for a couple of days. That was one of the few things I found frightening.

—Billie Chapin

The hospital became a cheerier place, too.

> *As everyone on this case was so low during the period of deepest coma because of our apparent inability to have any positive effect, the staff was tremendously buoyed by the first signs of improvement. The spirits of everyone just shot up.*
>
> —T. Scammell, MD

> *It seemed too good to be true. Maybe, I just couldn't believe it.*
>
> —Bruce

At the time, no one knew exactly how matters would play out, but the news was good, for a change, and the people around me dared to think it might continue.

◆ ◆ ◆

Medical Notes, Beth Israel-Deaconess

May 31, 1998

4:39 AM Intensive Care, progress note:

Extremities remain flaccid although patient continues to grimace and yawn. [She] appears to attempt to open her eyes when her name is called.

—F. E. Arlia, RN

1:13 PM Internal Medicine, off-service note:

Neurology: Contact plasmapheresis team if no dramatic improvement by tomorrow.

Social: Husband and mother are here daily. They are hopeful, but aware of the severity of her illness, uncertain recovery potential, and the need for extended rehabilitation … Will likely need several more days of observation, but will need to begin screening for rehab next week.

—M. McLaughlin, MD

6:48 PM Intensive Care, progress note:

Neurology: Patient attempting and, at times, able to open eyes upon request. Also once today, when eyes opened, patient smiled. Still no movement from extremities.

—E. M. Condon, RN

Neurology Consultant Attending.

Opens eyes to voice, follows one-step midline commands in fragmented fashion ["open/close your eyes," "open your mouth"]. Focused on examiner's face and smiled briefly. Had lengthy discussion with patient's husband this morning about diagnosis and prognosis. These will become clearer after several days.

—T. Scammell, MD

I had been on steroids for two days, and there was slight improvement. I fluttered my eyelids, and I moved my lips, slightly, as though I were attempting to speak. It might have seemed minimal, but improvements they were, and notable for their immediacy in response to the steroid therapy. But I was not yet out of danger.

The next day would be the first of June. On the first of every month at Beth Israel-Deaconess, rotations occur. My team was scheduled to be rotated off and a new team would come on board.

Bruce did not want this to happen. He did not want a group of new doctors coming on board, having to travel up the learning curve—he felt my case was just too complex. He explained the situation to Foster and together they appealed to the doctors to keep the team intact, at least until I stabilized.

Foster spoke with each of my doctors, including Dr. Saper, the chief of neurology, to back up the request. "I pushed all the institutional buttons I could," he would tell me later. "Something happened in that place twelve years ago—and I couldn't bear to have it happen again."

At the same time, Bruce met with Dr. Scammell in one of the ninth-floor conference rooms he was getting to know so well. "You and the other doctors who know the most about this rare case should not be disbanded," Bruce implored. "You must have a desire to learn more about the unusual nature of this disorder—why change hands while she's still in danger?

"Please, you just can't do it."

Dr. Scammell looked at Bruce for several moments. Then he agreed. Although it was a departure from normal Beth Israel-Deaconess procedure, the decision was made. My team would stay together to see me through.

♦ ♦ ♦

After twelve days in a coma, the last five of them on high-pulse doses of steroids, I began to regain consciousness. Little by little, I began my return. I opened my eyes, and, with the aid of my tracheostomy, I could talk, though only with difficulty and with great confusion. But I could talk.

My recovery, if it were to occur at all, would be from the top down. Due to the inflammation of my spinal cord, my limbs were extremely weak. I was, in fact, quadriplegic.

When I later studied my medical record, it was as though I were reading about another person. I was gratified to see the entries that made note of smiling, laughing, and joking. But I remember none of it; I was truly in another place that only God knows.

"It's actually very flattering," Dr. Scammell explained. "People with good spirits who recover from a serious injury will wake up laughing; the pleasant person becomes evident."

After all their trouble, my caregivers finally had an agreeable patient.

Medical Record, Beth Israel-Deaconess

June 1, 1998

5:35 AM Intensive Care, progress note:

Neuromuscular weakness: Upper and lower extremities remain flaccid. Patient ... opened her eyes when stimulated while being repositioned but did not open her eyes on command. Alteration to nutrition: ... Receiving tube feedings without incident.

—F. E. Arlia, RN

9:00 AM Neurology Consultant Attending:

Opens eyes to voice, clearly follows midline commands, smiles socially ... Though she grimaces rapidly to nail bed pressure, I can elicit no withdrawal of limbs ... Mental status improving nicely. Continue Solumedrol.

—T. Scammell, MD

1:38 PM Intensive Care Attending:

On pulse steroids over the weekend. Perhaps slight neuro improvement. Doing well on relatively small amount of ventilator support. No recent apneas witnessed ... Will try to arrange plasmapheresis today.

—R. M. Schwartzstein, MD

5:32 PM Internal Medicine, progress note:

... Forty-two-year-old female, well known to the MICU team, here with Acute Disseminated Encephalomyelitis, currently improving with high-dose steroids ... Was evaluated by plasmapheresis team today ... Transfusion medicine service feels that plasmapheresis may also help ... although given her improvement, not clear if she will still need it.

—D. M. Seo, MD

Rheumatology Fellow with Dr. Trentham:

Eyes open to hand squeeze, but still unresponsive to conversation ... We agree that the patchy white matter changes are more compatible with a diffuse encephalitis. Will sign off for now, but follow with interest the continuing infectious diseases and neurology evaluation.

—J. P. Whelan, MD, PhD

Social Work:

Patient's husband recognizes that patient's recuperation will be a lengthy process and that patient's potential is difficult for team to diagnose at this time. He is asking appropriate questions regarding rehabilitation facilities and would like information, which will be provided to him. [We] have also arranged for a psychologist to meet with patient's husband to address his questions and concerns regarding how to address patient's progress with their children.

—L. Cahey, Lic. SW

6:01 PM Intensive Care, progress note:

Much more responsive, even more so this evening. Looked toward speaker and laughed at a few jokes. Husband and mother in. Very encouraged by patient's responsiveness. Awaiting decision about plasmapheresis.

—J. A. Atterstrom, RN

On the evening of June 1, Foster visited me in the Intensive Care Unit. He was able to elicit an unusual reaction, perhaps the earliest sign of recognition in my subconscious state.

"I came to sit with you shortly after the steroids were started," Foster told me later. "Again, I didn't know what to say, or do. I just started talking about my attempt to build a dock up in Maine and my misadventures with the planning board. I thought it would help to talk about a place you know and love—the part of Maine we both know so well. You smiled and even gave a sort of odd little laugh."

Judy had witnessed the scene and was astonished that I not only seemed to recognize his voice, but that I also responded by smiling and attempting to laugh.

Apparently, it was the first instance of someone reaching me so early on.

Medical Record, Beth Israel-Deaconess

June 2, 1998

3:06 PM Intensive Care, progress note:

Patient not as alert during the early morning; later on, was much more alert, smiling at comments, able to follow commands during PE [physical exam]; still only moves the head ... Is currently doing well on trach mask. However, [patient] is requiring frequent suctions for increased secretions.

—D.M. Seo, MD

5:10 PM Intensive Care, progress note:

No movement below neck. Alert with periods of lethargy. Seems to understand some things, but cognition difficult to evaluate. Does not always follow commands. Grimaces when turned and when tape pulled off arm.

—J. A. Atterstrom, RN

5:45 PM Intensive Care Attending:

Has done well for the past 24 hours on a trach mask. Increasing level of consciousness ... On examination this afternoon, patient was awake and alert and responding to commands. Still unable to move extremities. This is the final day of high-dose steroids. Consider initiation of plasmapheresis tomorrow.

—R. M. Schwartzstein, MD

Neurology Consultant Attending:

[Patient is] alert, fixes, and follows well; smiles on command and left facial weakness is now only moderate. If she continues to improve at this rate, I feel that plasmapheresis will not be necessary ... Mr. Ford will try to track down Dr. Kanter so we can discuss ADEM and indications for plasmapheresis. Physical therapy should start working with her and please get her up to [a] chair as soon as possible.

—T. Scammell, MD

B.G. was thrilled and amazed that the steroids were working, but he expressed it as cautious optimism. He could see that I still was not moving, and always in the back of his mind was the uncertainty about the extent of my recovery—if it were to continue at all. He always wanted to keep one step ahead, but he was definitely heartened. He no longer had to think about his wife dying.

If the steroids had not worked, or if I had reached a plateau and stopped improving, the medical team most likely would have turned to plasmapheresis. This filtration process rids the blood of all potentially harmful antibodies, thus offering the same immune-suppressing potential as steroids.

Blood has two components, blood cells, red and white, and the fluid, or plasma, in which they travel. Dissolved in the plasma are antibodies.

Plasmapheresis separates the red blood cells from the plasma and returns them back into the blood stream—minus the harmful antibodies. A needle is inserted into one arm to withdraw the blood, which is then sent through a tube to a bedside filtration mechanism and returned to the bloodstream via a needle in the other arm. Filtration of a person's entire blood supply occurs over several days.

"It's quite a process," Dr. Scammell explained later, "and with hindsight, it might have been helpful. We considered trying it, but we were concerned that it could compromise the immune function. If this had been an infectious disease, plasmapheresis would have made things worse. It's a risky procedure."

Before the decision was made, Dr. Scammell and the rest of the team wanted to consult with Dr. Daniel Kanter of Brigham and Women's Hospital. Dr. Scammell had found several of Dr. Kanter's papers on ADEM to be of use early on. He also was known to have had some success with plasmapheresis. But Dr. Kanter had moved to an unknown location in the Midwest.

> *My goal was to get the doctors talking. I wanted to keep one step ahead of the game. One afternoon, I just took the phone to the hospital lobby and began calling. The first Cincinnati number I dialed was a wrong number, but the secretary of the company I had mistakenly dialed was able to tell me that Dr. Kanter's office was near Christ Hospital. When I called that hospital, I found out that Dr. Kanter was at a completely different location. It was as though he'd left Boston and didn't want to be found.*
>
> —Bruce

Ultimately, Bruce did obtain the correct number and faxed it to Dr. Scammell. In time, the doctors decided that plasmapherisis would not have to be undertaken.

But by then, there were further issues.

> *The other significant concern at that time was that the EEGs continued to show a slowing of the brain waves. We were still concerned about seizures. But there was hope. You had begun to follow what are considered to be complex commands. For example, closing your right eye on command, and not your left.*
>
> —T. Scammell, MD

So, knowing the difference between right and left was considered complex. How life changes. One of my last assignments before falling ill had been to write a speech for Foster to deliver in Tokyo on the globalization of the investment and pension business. Now, it was a big deal to know left from right.

Medical Record, Beth Israel-Deaconess

June 3, 1998

2:24 PM Internal Medicine, progress note:

After consulting with neurology and transfusion medicine, will hold off on plasmapheresis unless recovery plateaus or declines ... Patient to be rescreened for rehab placement, one that can keep a close eye on her neurologic status.

—D. M. Seo, MD

3:33 PM. Intensive Care, progress note:

Patient mouthing words [and] appears better as day progresses. Patient is alert, able to move head side to side and stick tongue out and smile. Neurology commented on right finger movement, which was not seen by this RN. Neurology states right upper extremity will be first extremity that will show improvement in mobility.

—T. E. Ledoux, RN

4:04 PM Intensive Care Attending:

Continues to do well on trach mask. Making progress on all fronts ... Disposition of rehab being assessed.

—R. M. Schwartzstein, MD

Neurology Consultant Attending:

Patient now alert and following more complex commands ... Flicker of movement in right finger flexors [tendons that allow fingers to bend] but still frankly quadriplegic. Can feel light touch in right upper extremity, less so in left upper extremity, probably no sensation in feet ... Please repeat EEG.

—T. Scammell, MD

I apparently woke up *trying*. My slurred speech was a concern. My inability to speak prompted people to wonder how the ultimate damage would affect my ability to communicate.

"It was disturbing to see the perfect communicator unable to speak well," Foster would tell me. "But you never fretted. You were always trying to enunciate every word, to do better—to *re*do."

Medical Record, Beth Israel-Deaconess

June 4, 1998

Neurology:

More alert today ... Mouthed several words today ... Remains unable to establish consistent communication ... Left facial drops ... Able to protrude tongue today ... No movement noted in extremities ... Will review EEG to plan Dilantin management.

—B. Murray, MD

Neurology Consultant Attending:

Improvement continues—mouthing long sentences, spoke briefly when trach tube changed yesterday, small movement of finger flexor [a tendon in the finger that allows it to move] ... with tiny movements of left toes. If she has difficulty speaking with trach, we might consider a translator for deaf patients, who can read lips.

—T. Scammell, MD

◆ ◆ ◆

My first lucid statement upon awakening was to my mother. It was also my first post-coma instruction, "Mom, Lindsay likes macaroni and cheese for lunch."

My first post-coma joke was with Cathy Ebling, who told me Hilly would be over soon to give me a big hug.

"No hanky-panky," said Mom.

In my best Tallulah Bankhead voice, I hoarsely whispered to Cathy, "Tell Hilly ... we can do hanky-panky."

When I asked Bruce where he was when I woke up and what words I first spoke to him, it took a while for me to understand that my questions did not apply. He wasn't there, because he could not bear it.

Judy's favorite story centered on my children. A mother herself, she easily imagined the effect of the long absence of a mother, even temporarily, on such young children. She was concerned about Westy and Lindsay and how they were making it through all that had happened. After I had made some progress regaining consciousness, she thought it would be good for my children to hear my voice.

One night, she called my home. "Bruce," she said, "I think Wendy might be able to talk to the kids tonight." Bruce screened me for my ability to speak. "I knew he would do that," Judy would later tell me.

Then he put Westy on the phone; Lindsay was already asleep. Although I retained no memory of this conversation, I was apparently able to speak coherently and, most importantly, lovingly to Westy. Judy told me I said all the right things.

"It's so good to hear your voice, Westy," I said, as Judy held the phone to my ear. "This is the best medicine I could ever have. I miss you so much. But the doctors are very, very good, and they're helping me get better. I love you. I miss you."

As I carried on my first conversation with my young son in weeks, tears began to stream down Judy's cheeks and those of the other nurses standing nearby. One might have thought that intensive care nurses were inured to such scenes, but apparently not. At Bruce's end, he was trying, successfully no doubt, to control his emotions for Westy's sake.

"It was an extraordinary evening," Judy later recalled.

I had a number of visitors and other telephone conversations shortly after I regained consciousness. I had a long talk on the phone with my brother, Kim, who called from Santa Fe, and I received visits from some of my favorite people. I still don't remember any of the conversations.

Clearly, I was also unable to fully appreciate or emotionally process what was going on. When Judy began to tell me the details of my medical adventure, I reacted as if I were at a social occasion listening to someone else's story. I didn't seem to be the least bit distraught.

"Oh, my goodness," I said in the best conversational manner. "You don't say ... Oh, my ... how awful."

Even after I began to make further progress and was able to speak more coherently, Judy was often puzzled by some of the things I said.

You were always articulate and polite, and you made a lot of sense. But there were times when I just couldn't fully comprehend what you were saying. At first, I thought you were talking above me intellectually because you were so well spoken—and you didn't seem confused. But then I started to ask questions about exactly what you had said, and I realized you weren't quite altogether there. Everything seemed logical up to a point, but a couple of your words would always be off. You would start a story, and it would make perfect sense—except for a couple of zingers at the end that just didn't fit.

—J. A. Atterstrom, RN

For example, I began one conversation by saying, "The doctors came in yesterday, and they were so nice, but they didn't bring their credit cards!"

Others remembered being struck by my entrenched manners. With purposeful formality, I was apparently determined to make the acquaintance of everyone who came into my room to attend to me.

"Now, what is your name?" I would ask pleasantly.

"Mary," was one response. "Mary Smith."

"Oh ... Mary Smith ... Very nice."

Then I would continue to address the person by name, I suppose because it seemed the right thing to do, despite my general confusion. Perhaps I did it just to get a better hold on my new surroundings or to exercise my mind. With my spotty memory, it was an obvious challenge.

◆　◆　◆

Medical Record, Beth Israel-Deaconess

June 4, 1998

5:38 PM Intensive Care Attending:

Patient had one episode of desaturation last night that cleared with suctioning. Continues to do well on trach mask. On exam this morning, patient was awake and alert ... Patient able to make slight movement of fingers ... [There is] slow ongoing improvement off steroids. Respiratory status stable ... Clearly will need long rehab stay.

—R. M Schwartzstein, MD

5:43 PM Intensive Care, progress note:

She is able to interact, nod appropriately. Slight movement of fingers and toes to command. Seen by physical therapist; out of bed to chair for 3 hours. Patient does seem to be slightly confused/forgetful. Unable to state husband's name or where she lives.

—R. Griggs, RN

5:51 PM Intensive Care, progress note:

Husband spoke with social services regarding rehab options. Team feels that patient will be ready to transfer in the next few days.

—R. Griggs, RN

Again, B.G. did extensive research, this time to determine the best place for me to be transferred for rehabilitation. He was relieved that I had been saved but wary about the uncertain prospects for my recovery. He was always thinking, preparing, always being thorough. Representatives from rehab hospitals were in abundance at acute-care hospitals such as Beth Israel-Deaconess. There was no shortage of information or pitches. But we were fortunate to have an objective resource—a friend who heads a hospital north of Boston. When asked to rate the several facilities Bruce had researched, he declared without hesitation that "Spaulding is a ten." That was all he needed to hear.

Spaulding Rehabilitation Hospital had an affiliation with Massachusetts General Hospital and Harvard Medical School that also worked in its favor, as did its location in Boston, just a few miles north of Beth Israel-Deaconess. The threshold for getting me back to the Beth Israel-Deaconess Medical Center in an emergency had to be very low. Bruce was assured that a transfer could be done within fifteen minutes, if necessary. Thus, the decision to admit me to Spaulding was made with great confidence. It was a decision that would prove to be rewarding in ways that could never be measured in any conventional sense.

Medical Record, Beth Israel-Deaconess

June 5, 1998

11:33 AM Radiology, final report:

Assess for pneumonia. There is a tracheostomy tube in place, unchanged from prior films. The lungs are clear, showing no evidence of pneumonia ... The cardiac silhouette and vascular markings are normal. Conclusion: No evidence of pneumonia.

—R. A. Kane, MD

Neurology:

Alert. Following commands—gave husband's name when asked, responded appropriately to questions ... Moved both feet a trace when asked ...

Continued improvement several days off steroids. Taper Dilantin off ... If seizure occurs, or suspicion, would reload Dilantin.

—B. Murray, MD

Neurology Attending:

Agree with Dilantin taper.

—T. Scammell, MD

Social Work:

Patient screened by Spaulding and clinically accepted. (This is family's first choice at present.)

—L. Cahey, Lic. SW

3:00–4:00 PM Occupational Therapy, evaluation:

Patient [is] lethargic. Follows simple commands ... Mouthing words but unable to speak ... Appears aware of situation. Repeating, "I'm missing my kids."

Medical Record, Beth Israel-Deaconess

June 6, 1998

5:33 AM Intensive Care, progress note:

[Patient is] alert and interactive; able to wiggle toes of left foot. No movement of upper extremities noted tonight, but has been able to move fingers on previous shift. Secretions increased [but] no acute distress noted.

—P. A. Chabre, RN

3:02 PM Internal Medicine, progress note:

Patient reports no pain, breathing comfortably ... Current issue includes temperature spikes with unknown source.

—D. M. Seo, MD

Medical Record, Beth Israel-Deaconess

June 7, 1998

5:33 AM Intensive Care, progress note:

Patient is animated and jokes ... Once told the correct answers, she gives the accurate information back. Extremities are not moving, but [she] pulls away from painful stimuli.

—C. J. Perella, RN

Neurology Attending:

Awake and alert in chair. Clenches left more than right fist; moves left toes more than right. Some good orientation. She said, "You are Dr. Walsh or Dr. Scammell" without prompting. Other times confused: "You helped me with the French restaurant." She still has fevers.

—C. Walsh, MD

Medical Record, Beth Israel-Deaconess

June 8, 1998

6:41 AM Intensive Care, progress note:

Intermittently is A&Ox3. [Alert and oriented times three. The patient knows #1 WHO she is; #2 WHERE she is; #3 WHAT the date is. Sometimes I answered questions correctly, and sometimes not, i.e., a bit "off," but not completely confused. According to Judy, sometimes when patients are A&Ox3, they are just lucky to get the answers right. Other times, they memorize the answers after being asked "a zillion times a day," but that, in itself, is a good sign.] Other times, she confabulates a story based on something that did happen over the past several weeks while [she was] here at Beth Israel-Deaconess.

—C. J. Perella, RN

12:35 PM Intensive Care, transfer note:

Patient has a very supportive family: husband, two children (ages three and eight years), and a mother ... Patient should be going to Spaulding Rehab sometime this week. Also, it was mentioned in rounds that before the patient leaves the hospital, the trach might be replaced with a fenestrated trach [this enables a small amount of air to pass through the trach, allowing the patient to speak].

—E. M. Condon, RN

Social Work:

Contacted by Spaulding this afternoon with financial precertification and bed offer when patient is medically stable ... Have discussed with patient's family, who are aware and in agreement with plans for transfer.

—L. M. Pleasance, PT

Neurology Attending:

[Patient] feels well; no complaints. In fact, seems to neglect the severity of her deficits, though she hears her named paged ... Continues to make excellent daily progress, though quadriplegia is slow to improve ... Will consider transfer to Spaulding if she remains stable for one or two [more] days.

—T. Scammell, MD

I remember nothing before June 8, my last full day at Beth Israel-Deaconess. My memories of that day are sketchy and disjointed, but at least I have them. It was my forty-third birthday, and a number of people came to visit. Everyone smiled cheerfully, which was very brave of them all, for I was obviously quadriplegic—could hardly move a thing—and it wasn't apparent if I ever would again. Everyone was aware of the uncertainty. Mostly, I remembered Westy hopping around in his artsy Eric Hopkins tee shirt from Maine, with the big lobster claw on the front, and thinking that the design was vaguely familiar.

> *You were awake. Hilly Ebling and several of your friends from John Hancock were there. You were not able to use your muscles, but you were smiling and talking as well as you could. Your room was filled with flowers. Westy was so glad to see you. You were able to talk a little and touch him. I think it helped him to be able to see you and know that even though you were ill, you still loved him.*
>
> —Billie Chapin

◆ ◆ ◆

And so I survived. Apparently it was amazing that I did. The doctors could not fully explain it. Certainly, the administration of high-dose pulse steroids for five days had an effect. But steroid therapy was not always successful in such cases, and the doctors weren't sure it would work for me. Dr. Trentham, the rheumatologist, considered the possibility that Doxycycline, which was administered for several days, perhaps had a serendipitous effect. Doxycycline was a safe antibiotic with anti-inflammatory properties. It was commonly used to treat acne and also rheumatoid arthritis, the latter for its ability to reduce inflammation of the joints. It was prescribed for me because of its ability to counter nitric oxide, the chemical made by white blood cells that amplifies inflammation. But whether Doxycycline had any positive effect has remained a medical uncertainty.

◆ ◆ ◆

Although I had, indeed, survived, a huge problem loomed. My central nervous system had been attacked. I had a brain and spinal cord disorder and was quadriplegic. To one degree or another, it affected nearly all of my capabilities, mental and physical. Although I smiled a lot, perhaps I just didn't understand.

"I remember being struck by the contrast between your cheeriness and your situation," Dr. Scammell would relate.

And again, because there were so few recorded incidences of ADEM, reliable prognostication for my rehabilitation was impossible. Bruce was given little reason for hope or optimism. Shortly after I emerged from the coma, one of the doctors told my husband, "She might *begin* to show some progress by Christmas."

Still, he was greatly relieved; he no longer believed that I would die. His worst fear had been having to tell the children that their mother had not survived, and then, parenting alone in grief. We had been such a great team for those kids.

Yet no one could predict to what extent my physical and cognitive ability would return. Would it be 10 percent—or 50 percent? Would I be impaired for the rest of my life? Would I be in a wheelchair? Would I be able to look after my children? Or would I have to live in an assisted-care facility away from my family? These were shattering questions to ponder.

For the moment, June 8, 1998, only one thing was certain. Dr. Scammell and his troops at Beth Israel-Deaconess had defied seemingly insurmountable odds.

"The reason I went into neurology was the mystery," Dr. Scammell explained to me later. "The truth is that we have a very superficial understanding of the brain. We really don't know that much about how it works, and that was one of the attractions. Your case was right up there. We worked very, very hard—and we were still baffled. Seeing someone make such a dramatic recovery can help promote one's commitment to working hard, digging deep, trying to find the answers. I frequently use your story when I interview residents—to see whether they're quitters."

Thank God Dr. Scammell wasn't a quitter.

Part Two

"She will probably remain quadriplegic indefinitely."

Dr. Joel Stein, June 1998
Spaulding Rehabilitation Hospital
Boston, Massachusetts

Chapter Four

Out of the Fire

June 9, 1998, the day of my transfer to Spaulding Rehabilitation Hospital, the weather was sunny and humid. The ambulance trip across my beautiful city, which I barely recognized from that vantage point, was bumpy and warm. I felt a bit in limbo. I did not know what to expect and oddly, perhaps, I was unconcerned. Most likely, I was unable to process emotionally what was happening and, therefore, incapable of worry. It felt as though I were going from one cocoon to another. I had no doubt that I would be well cared for.

The solicitous ambulance attendants hovered over me. "Are you comfortable?" one asked. "It's not too warm, is it?"

I realized that it was almost summertime, my favorite season. This was the time for tennis, sailing, long vacations in Maine, and playing on the beach and swimming with my children. It all seemed so far away, like a dream. I remember thinking, "I have to get back there, to Maine." The light was so bright that morning. It was nice to be out in the air and to see the sunshine.

At my new hospital, I was wheeled in through a side entrance and brought to the fourth floor, a stroke floor. I wondered, "How long will I be here? How long will it take?" I saw Bruce and Mom waiting for me, brave little smiles on their faces, trying their best to look cheery and hopeful. "Oh, good," I remember thinking. "They're here." I was the youngest patient in that section of the hospital, by far. "But what am I doing here? How did I get to this? What happened?" On the day of my admission to Spaulding, my ELOS (estimated length of stay) was twelve weeks.

Much later, Sally Frank, the wife of my next-door hospital neighbor, Dr. Howard Frank, told me, "We were devastated to see such a young person so gravely ill arrive that day. The breathing apparatus and all the IV tubes. It was a sight."

While my cognitive abilities and sense of self-awareness were significantly diminished, I fervently believe it was all for the best. It was also fortunate that I was unable to see myself. Amazingly, I was not upset.

My primary physician at Spaulding was Dr. Joel Stein. In addition to teaching at Harvard Medical School, he was the director of Stroke Rehabilitation at Spaulding. He cared for individuals with a variety of neurologic conditions that included multiple sclerosis and Parkinson's disease. Dr. Paul Sandhu was one of my attending physicians. Both physicians were as puzzled about the cause of my illness and uncertain about my potential for recovery, just as my team of doctors at Beth Israel-Deaconess had been.

"In the literature, there are few cases of ADEM, and their causes are poorly understood," Dr. Sandhu later wrote me. "Your case was quite puzzling … and your thorough evaluation revealed no clues as to what initiated the downward spiral [and] eventual paralysis."

Not only was the condition rare, it had a great variance in recovery. It was not possible to identify the percentage of ADEM patients who recovered at all, let alone fully. It was virtually impossible to prognosticate with any accuracy; the doctors were pessimistic.

Shortly after I arrived, Dr. Stein responded to Dr. Sandhu's query about my potential for recovery by replying, "She will probably remain quadriplegic indefinitely."

Later, Dr. Stein wrote me, saying, "On a personal level, it is always difficult to be confronted with someone with major neurological limitations, and this is amplified when the patient is young, intelligent, and has a family with young children. Nonetheless, we are in the hope business, and I try to look at the positive aspects of every patient's situation …"

I loved that phrase, "the hope business," because hope was just about all that I had.

◆ ◆ ◆

At Spaulding Rehab, they quickly came to know me.

None of us—not Bruce, nor Mom, nor I—knew what to expect from a rehab hospital. I've since come to realize that most people don't know about rehab hospitals until they become a patient in one. From the start, as I had done at Beth Israel-Deaconess, I made a point of learning as many names as possible. I felt that I had the best of everything at Spaulding and of everyone—doctors, nurses, and therapists. I felt they deserved to be addressed by name. It was also a sort of intellectual goal, one more thing to work on and see whether I could master it.

In another burst of great fortune for me, Teresa McLaughlin was assigned to be my primary nurse at Spaulding. When I arrived, she was about to dive into a slice of pizza at a birthday party for another nurse. Her supervisor stopped her.

"Don't even pick that up," she warned Teresa. "A very sick woman has just arrived from Beth Israel, and she's yours."

Teresa came over as I was being wheeled into my room.

"Please," I croaked in a voice that was weak but imploring, "Could I have some Evian water?"

Pas possible. Had I been able to swallow anything, let alone Evian, Teresa might have gotten a kick out of my request. But because of the trach, I couldn't. I was fed and administered medications and liquid through the PEG tube in my stomach. If I had drunk Evian, or anything else, through my mouth, I would have begun to drown. I do remember being so very thirsty and wanting terribly much to brush my teeth.

Bruce took Teresa aside right away on another matter.

"You know," he whispered to her out of my earshot, "she washes her hair every day. Is there something you can do? She would flip if she saw how she looked right now."

"I'll give her a shower every morning," Teresa promised, even though it took three people, including the strong, young aide, Constantine, to get me out of bed and into the big waterproof wheelchair.

But it was worth it. Those showers were refreshingly humanizing. Teresa also bought some nice shampoo for me to replace the standard hospital issue, and Mom imported my favorite French soap and Chanel No. 5. These were small steps toward normalcy.

In the first week of my stay at Spaulding, I had a couple of VIP visits. Bruce brought Westy and Lindsay to see me. It had been about one month since I had seen my daughter. She was wearing a pretty purple dress that her Aunt Anne had sent from Santa Fe. Lindsay, who was a real spark plug, seemed unusually quiet, almost distant. Because I could not move my arms, I was unable to hug her.

"B.G.," I asked, "can you just set her on the bed, right next to me, so that I can at least be touching her?"

While I remembered this scene afterward, somehow I could not fully process its poignancy. I remember feeling unable to do what I wanted, which was to hug my children. But I was not in despair. I was so glad to see them, especially Lindsay. Bruce hadn't brought her to Beth Israel-Deaconess. He thought it would be too frightening for her, and he wasn't sure how well I would be able to converse. But even though Lindsay was now at Spaulding, the question remained. What was the effect of my drastically changed appearance on this young girl not yet three and one-half years old?

After a while, I tuckered out and the visit came to an end. Weeks later, Teresa, a spirited, young, native Bostonian, told me the visit was more than *she* could bear. She was so distraught by my inability to hug the children, she went home and cried all weekend.

Teresa stories abound. We had a great time together, joking and gabbing about the various personalities around the hospital. She was always so attentive to my children, both of whom took to her immediately. I'm sure that it was good for Westy and Lindsay to see that someone so wonderful was taking care of their mom. I began to think of Teresa as the fun little sister I never had.

"How *ahh* you this morning?" Teresa would ask in her great Boston accent as she made her way down our hall. Smiles appeared instantly. She looked like a young Elizabeth Taylor, bursting with energy. She had spirit and spunk to spare. Somehow, she managed to impart her good will and vibrant personality without fooling those of us in our unfortunate circumstances. It was her great gift. She lifted the spirits of everyone on the fourth floor of Spaulding Rehab.

Chapter Five

Impossible Memories

I brought some strangely vivid memories with me to Spaulding. I say "brought" because I had them from the beginning of my stay, yet I don't necessarily remember them as originating there. Unlike dreams, these imaginings were as vivid and realistic as memories of actual occurrences. But it would have been impossible for them to occur, given my profound physical limitations.

One memory is of waiting in a family restaurant in the lobby of Beth Israel-Deaconess. But there is no such place at Beth Israel. And, of course, it would have been impossible for me to get there by myself. Wait staff in striped shirts and baseball caps whizzed by. Everyone ignored me. I don't remember any other people being in the restaurant, which was dimly lit. I do remember that somehow I had arranged for balloons for my children and a luscious cake with lots of whipped cream for dessert. I kept thinking about how much they would enjoy all the arrangements I was making for them.

At the same time, a sale was being held to benefit a charity. I remember buying a number of items for Westy and Lindsay. There was a stroller with a teddy bear design that I thought Lindsay would like. "Would it fit at our table?" I remembered wondering. I also remember having a hard time operating the portable phone at my table. "Why won't this work?" I wondered. "It's 6:00 PM. B.G. must know I'm here, that I'm waiting. How could he not know that I'm here?" I tried to reach him repeatedly, but had no success. I remember waiting, puzzled and frustrated that my family was not there, and wanting desperately to see my children.

But they never came.

In another memory, I was in an art gallery much like Pierre Deux. Apparently, it was adjacent to Beth Israel-Deaconess—another distinct impossibility. The actual Pierre Deux is in another part of Boston and several miles away on Newbury Street. I remember that one of my doctors, young and sandy-haired much like Dr. Scammell and wearing a white coat, was involved in the ownership of the gallery—only it was not Dr. Scammell.

The doctor appeared in the gallery. I considered some things to buy. Tired, I sat on a divan.

"You will be taken care of," said the young man in the white coat.

I examined some tall candlesticks. They were yellow and blue, typical country French style, and rather expensive. I vacillated before deciding to purchase them.

"Oh, Tim would love these," I thought, remembering my great friend from John Hancock. "The cost be damned!"

I later recounted this episode to my friend Kimberly Patton. A professor at Harvard Divinity School, she was working on a book on comparative religion. She spoke of out-of-body experiences, the writing and research being done on the subject, the mystery—as well as the possibility—of it all.

"That's very interesting," I said, hearing her out. "But it's all kind of *unbelievable*, isn't it?"

"Maybe," she said with an impish grin, "you just went shopping!"

A couple of weeks later, after Bruce had begun to pay my bills, he walked into my room and joked about appropriating my American Express card.

"I'd like to see that bill," I said, in all seriousness. "I think there are some things on it that I haven't taken delivery of … and it isn't right, taking advantage of a sick woman."

There were other impossible memories. I was asked to make an appearance at a benefit fundraiser for the hospital. It included a snowy drive into New Hampshire. (On the Spaulding Turnpike, perhaps?) I remember being briefed on my role and feeling extremely weak. Hilly and Cathy figured prominently in this image, buying gifts for the children at the event. Perhaps I was subconsciously remembering earlier ski weekends with our great friends. Or, perhaps I sensed, at some level, how well they were entertaining my family.

"This is the hardest thing that you will ever have to do," one of the organizers told me, a sentiment that could apply fittingly to what I was about to undertake at Spaulding Rehab.

I also had a "memory" of a weekend outside London in a country house. The weather was cold and chilly, fly-fishing was the order of the day, and Dr. Scammell was in attendance. I hadn't been to London in years, and I don't fish. Very strange.

Other memories took me to a diverse number of places including a marine biology laboratory somewhere much like Bermuda (another of my favorite destinations). I had a memory of the intrigue in the Santa Fe art dealers' world and examining Native American art and artifacts, which was exactly what I did when I visited there. I also experienced a memory of getting around on a rainy night in Boston and being delayed. Unsure of my destination, I was thinking that my brother would meet me at some point. I ended up in an old townhouse much like the one Bruce and I lived in years earlier, in Boston's Back Bay. The memories often were very dark and always very confusing.

"How could I have done these things?" I asked Teresa. I was puzzled and clearly adrift. "Would it have been possible?"

"I don't think so," she murmured, shaking her head with a barely concealed look of concern. At that juncture, she might have wondered whether I had problems in addition to the quadriplegia.

Another compelling memory was especially mysterious and disturbing because it was recurring; I was never quite sure what it meant. It began with my being driven down a highway at night. The glare of headlights illuminated signs indicating that we were driving through Kentucky, destination unknown. It seemed like a twilight zone. My driver, a young, clean-cut fellow and muscular, wore a gray tee-shirt imprinted with USMC in large capital letters. He resembled no one I knew and was completely unfamiliar to me. He said nothing, but he looked determined and concerned. Curiously, I was not frightened. I clearly remember sitting in the seat on the passenger side and looking over at him, wondering why he was concentrating so hard, wondering where we were going. No words were exchanged. The ride seemed to last forever.

Later, I was tempted to wonder if my young driver was a messenger of some sort, dispatched to usher me to another place, but experiencing second thoughts. He seemed sure of his role, but there was deep uncertainty about our ultimate destination.

In another sequence, I remember being at a school or another institutional setting—perhaps a hospital—where food and cakes were made with IV supplies. I remember the smell of the place, it was rather sweet and stuffy in a sort of clinical way. Perhaps it was the way the hospital smelled to my unconscious self. Again, there was the waiting—always the feeling of interminable waiting—for rides and for people who never appeared. Perhaps that was what happened to a borderline Type A personality, which I certainly was, rendered comatose. Impatience was bound to persist—even at the subconscious level.

Of course, hidden messages and double meanings abounded throughout these "memories." And nearly every one of them, I came to realize, centered on one of my coma sitters. Perhaps they had gotten through to me.

The final strange, but perhaps understandable, memory I experienced early at Spaulding centered on trying to imagine how it would be for me when I returned home. How would I get around? But when I thought of home, I conjured scenes of my childhood home in Michigan, rather than my present home in Massachusetts.

Dr. Wayne Klein, Spaulding's neuropsychologist, suggested, "The memories might have something to do with the effect of the steroids or with the near-death experience."

It was the first time I had heard anyone use the phrase "near death" to describe my situation.

Chapter Six

"Pleasant, but confused"

The baseline personality observation on my Spaulding medical record, "pleasant, but confused," was true. I was determined. But, at least in the beginning, I was deluded as well. I never thought of myself as a quadriplegic. Bruce and my clinicians were unfailingly gentle about this, playing along with my delusions as though I were a child. The focus was on getting me better, physically and mentally—if possible—but always with compassion. Whenever I did try to understand at some level, my mental defenses must have kicked in, to help me evade the truth. Although I seemed to ignore my impairment, I had one persistent thought from the beginning of my return to consciousness that belied my lack of awareness: I wanted to be back in Maine with my family. After all, it was summertime.

The first time I had set foot in Maine, with B.G., decades earlier, I fell in love with it. The hills, the cool night air, the evergreens along the water's edge, and the islands off the rugged, rocky coast were all breathtakingly beautiful. It reminded me of my favorite childhood places back home on the Great Lakes, places such as Harbor Springs in northern Michigan and Port Elgin in Ontario, where I went in summer. As a transplanted Midwesterner, Maine was very special to me. From the beginnings of consciousness and memory on the last day of my stay at Beth Israel-Deaconess, I thought about returning to Maine, where my family and I had spent every summer for decades.

My first thought was of our old camp behind the Camden Hills at Tilden Pond. And for a person in my condition, the overarching question was: "How will I get to the water?"

I tried to figure out how I could navigate the way from our cabin down to the dock. I remembered thinking that it was good that the camp was on one level. I probably could be placed in the old red canoe to get out on the water without too much trouble. I imagined that I could be paddled around to see the sights, perhaps even visit friends down the lake and enjoy the loons. *Who knows?* I thought. *Perhaps I can even get* into *the water.*

And so I had this fortuitous and distinct visualization regarding my memory of and desire to return to Maine. But rather than visualizing the beautiful view looking out from the camp, what I saw in my mind's eye was a vision of myself walking away from the camp, across the lawn, and down to the dock. It was as though I were watching myself from the dock. This was long before anyone had the slightest notion that I would ever walk again. This image was not consciously summoned; it occurred to me naturally, early on in my rehab career. I later wondered if it might have been my willpower starting to crank up. In retrospect, it seems like a mysterious gift.

But then I remembered that we no longer went to Tilden Pond.

Wait, I thought, *we don't own the camp any more. But we still go to Maine …*

I know it. There's another place, but where?

It wouldn't come to mind right away, and I was so puzzled. But after a mental struggle that seemed to take days, the memory of the right place finally did come back. For years after we sold the camp, we took the month of July at a charming old farmhouse known as the Foote House, on the St. George peninsula. When the Foote House came into focus in my mind's eye, my first thought again was daunting: those steep captain's stairs to the second floor. I remembered the winding path through the meadow to the water. I also envisioned the steps and steep ramp down to the dock. Again, I had problems to solve.

How am I going to deal with those stairs? I thought, perplexed. *How am I going to get to the water? Especially at low tide?*

I never thought of myself as quadriplegic. However, I must have realized, at some level, the seriousness of my physical situation and the uncertain prospects looming before me. A mental defense must have set in that enabled me to turn away from the reality of my impairment and avoid becoming discouraged, in order to withstand the hard work that lay ahead.

I was fortunate that my cognitive abilities of memory and self-awareness, though seriously diminished, would return at approximately the same rate as my physical ability. Perhaps that enabled me to stay cheerful during rehab. One small indication of my confusion was that I kept calling Teresa, whom I saw several times a day, virtually every day, Genevieve. And I've never been able to conjure the name that I came up with for Constantine, the aide, only that it was wrong and very odd. Constantine, my gentle helper, never corrected me; he just knew when I was asking for him.

◆ ◆ ◆

Friends and acquaintances had different first impressions of my situation at Spaulding. When my friend Molly Ettenborough came to visit, she was distraught. She kept her feelings to herself at the time, but she later told me that the first thing that occurred to her was, "My God, Wendy can't move anything!"

She brought some photographs with her to share. "Here are the children at our Halloween party last year," she explained, as she searched my eyes for a flicker of recognition. "Here we all are on the boat at Steep Hill Beach last summer in Ipswich. Do you remember?"

"Oh, thank you," I said, vaguely, politely, weakly. "That's nice ..." Inwardly, I was still out in left field. I did not remember.

But old pals Sally and Jim Fitzpatrick saw something else. "We didn't know what to expect," Sally later explained, "but we were so inspired that you were 'all there.' You were articulate; your idiom, your humor and personality, were all there. We were walking on air when we left."

"At your core, despite all that had happened," said Jane Philippi, another friend from John Hancock, "There was this nice, *nice* person at your core. It was impressive."

But why was she so surprised, I wondered!

I was uncomfortable accepting the accolades about my attitude during this medical adventure. There was no alternative but to be positive. It wasn't as though I declared that I would be the cheerful stoic. It was fairly clear. At some basic level, I simply understood that I had so much work to do that I couldn't possibly expend energy on anything that would get in my way—especially anything negative. It never occurred to me to be bitter or to wallow in self-pity. Also, I've never enjoyed disappointing people, so how could I not appreciate the incredible efforts that were being mounted on my behalf by my doctors, therapists, and my tribe of family and friends to help bring me back?

People asked, "Why Wendy?"

My thought on that notion never wavered. "Why not?" We're all human beings, and things like this happen. It's as simple as that.

From the beginning of my stay at Spaulding, my focus was to gain the physical strength I would need to accomplish the Herculean task of recovery. The mental strength, the *will*, was there. I may have been confused, but I was nothing, if not determined.

This had become my work, my occupation. I was no longer a mother, except in my heart. I certainly was no longer a speechwriter. My eyes were hypersensitive to light, making it difficult to read, and, of course, there was no way I could have manipulated any sort of writing instrument, be it a pen or computer. And despite what Sally and Jim thought, I wasn't "all there." Though getting better, I was still loopy. My new career was to make myself whole again.

Determination was a huge factor. On that point, I will claim credit. I was extraordinarily determined, more so than at any other time in my life. There was no alternative except to do my personal best at this most difficult physical undertaking of my life. Elizabeth Campbell Martin is my first real friend, dating to Sunday school at the First Presbyterian Church in Bay City, Michigan, in the late 1950s. She wrote me on June 16, two days after we had talked on the telephone:

Dear Wendy,

It was so good to hear your voice on Sunday! We are glad to hear you are improving every day. Your dear mother and wonderful husband Bruce have kept us abreast of your health changes—we're always happy to hear of progress! I know you have work ahead to regain your movement and strength, but you can do it! You are my most determined friend (and that helps!) …

Love,

Elizabeth

People remembered my "working like fury," as Foster would put it, and they were absolutely right. It was daunting for family and friends to observe seemingly minute triumphs. For example, I was proud of my ability to raise my arms. This apparently simple task took me days to accomplish! I remembered the moment I got my arms in the air. It was a triumph, and I was excited about the promise of more progress. I knew I could do it; I *had* to do it. I had to exercise my body as much as I could by moving any little thing that would move, over and over and *over* again.

"Mrs. Ford's awake," the nurses joked. "Even though we can't see her face, her toes are wiggling; her feet are moving back and forth."

In the beginning, that was about all that I could move.

It was impossible for me to imagine anyone being more determined to win back a life. It was hard to think of anyone with so much to live for not being similarly determined. I'd had such a rich, full life: two beautiful children, a fabulous and devoted husband, and an incredible network of family, friends, and colleagues. I had an interesting career with an excellent company and worked for a prince of an individual. I was fortunate in so many ways.

I had so much to reclaim.

Chapter Seven

To Get Back Home

If a runner in the Boston Marathon can make it past Heartbreak Hill, the series of four rises that terminates five miles from the end of the 26.2-mile race, he or she is home free—physically and mentally. My Heartbreak Hill was the challenge of walking again. From the beginning of my rehab career, my goal, as impossible as it seemed, was to walk out of Spaulding Hospital with my family and not leave in a wheelchair. Physical, occupational, and speech and language pathology therapists worked with me daily.

Dawn Lucier was my primary physical therapist and a perfect choice because she was tough, exacting, and creative. She pushed me and took chances, experimenting and trying things that might have seemed overly ambitious or downright unrealistic. But I relished the challenges she set before me. In fact, I thirsted for them.

"I thought first about what I would need to do," she would say, recalling her first visit to my room, "and what equipment I'd have to get, such as a wheelchair and a sliding board, for transfers, for moving you to and from the chair.

"From there, my next thought was to see that you got the help you needed to do things, to complete each task we were asking of you. I remembered hearing your goal: to get back home.

"We didn't want to diminish hope. On the other hand, I would rather err on the side of caution and decrease hope, rather than raise false hopes. When you came in, you couldn't move anything other than your wrists and elbows, and those only minimally. We still didn't know why you had the disease. And because the disease was so rare, there was not a lot of research to allow us to prognosticate reliably. Nobody knew. Your prognosis and rehab potential were guarded."

I began my rehab career by flopping over in a wheelchair. It took the efforts of Dawn and two other therapists to transfer me from my bed to the chair. The sliding board, a smooth piece of wood approximately eight by twenty-four inches, was not my favorite item. The therapists used it to move me—slide me—between the wheelchair and the bed or onto a raised mat in the gym. It always hurt some part of my sore, atrophied body to be transferred, and it always seemed awkward and inconvenient. Once I was transferred to the wheelchair, a therapist put a seat belt around my waist to keep me from falling over. Then they wheeled me down to the fourth-floor gymnasium. It overlooked the Charles River and the extraordinary city of Boston with all of its old-world beauty and charm and its genius in the medical, educational, and financial arenas. It was a glorious, sparkling view with bright sunlight dancing on the water.

It also served as a constant, daily reminder of my former life.

To begin the session, the therapists propped me up on a raised mat by a wall of windows overlooking the Charles. It took two of them to hold me steady so that I wouldn't fall over. The third therapist worked with me. The first task the therapists set before me was curious. They put a large, slate-covered box on my lap and sprinkled it with talcum powder. They placed my arms on it and directed me to slide my arms over its surface as best I could.

As a former competitive tennis player, I was initially puzzled by these activities. I wondered how such simple movements could add up to anything of significance. What was going to happen? This won't amount to a hill of beans, I thought. Is this the right thing to do? Will it be enough? Do they know what they're doing?

Despite its minimal nature, this therapy was incredibly arduous in the early days, and weeks. I was not strong. I had lost 15 pounds from a 125-pound frame and was seriously impaired. My muscles had atrophied.

But I had to get better. There was no alternative.

One day, after you had just started your therapy, Bruce and I went down to the gym to watch. It was hard, because you were sort of like a Raggedy Annie. Your muscles couldn't hold you up, and often you would slump over, and say "Oops," and smile. It brought tears to my eyes. Bruce sat across the room and looked so despondent.

—Billie Chapin

Dawn explained what had to happen if I were ever to walk again. "In order to walk, you first have to learn to sit with balance," she said. "Then you have to be able to stand with balance. Only then can we start to work on the walking."

I didn't know how I would accomplish that, only that I would—that I must. At a point when my trunk musculature was still so impaired that

I couldn't even sit up straight without flopping over, I posed a question to Dawn. "What are my chances," I asked, half-embarrassed, looking up at her as I slumped over, "of getting out of here without this wheelchair?"

She spoke to me as one would to a child. "Well," she said. "It's kind of early. We'll see."

◆ ◆ ◆

June 15, 1998, Physician's progress notes:

Neurology:

Steady gains continue. Pulmonary: Trach removal today.

—J. Stein, MD

Feels well and made good progress by all accounts … Await HIV and other serologic.

—C. Hay, MD

◆ ◆ ◆

The doctors at Spaulding were aware of everything that had been tested at Beth Israel-Deaconess, but they did not necessarily know what had been contemplated. Thus, Dr. Stein, with Dr. Sandhu and Teresa standing by, told Bruce, "There is one test we haven't done."

Aware of our solid family history, the doctors suggested the topic they were broaching was unlikely to apply in my case "…unless of course, she's had a transfusion."

The test was for HIV, the same test that had been considered at Beth Israel-Deaconess but never carried out because I was unable to give consent. This test was yet another hammer-blow Bruce would have to endure.

When I had hemorrhaged following Westy's birth in July 1990, I lost 20 percent of my blood. Because I was so concerned about contracting the AIDS virus then, I wanted to avoid the transfusion. But I had to go through with it. My hematocrit, which refers to the proportion of blood cells to a volume of blood, should have been in the high thirties; mine had dropped to thirteen, too dangerously low to ignore.

"When do I have to decide?" I remember asking my obstetrician-gynecologist, Dr. David Hagen.

He gave me a rueful, little laugh and responded by telling me a story. "Just months ago, a young man in his twenties lost a tremendous amount of blood in a car accident," said Dr. Hagen. "He, too, vacillated about a transfusion for the same reasons you are, the fear of AIDS. He went into cardiac arrest right here in the hospital, but was too weak to survive it. His hematocrit was about the level of yours right now." He paused before adding, "You really don't have a lot of time to decide."

So the decision in 1990 was up to me, but I had no choice. Still, even though the blood supply was well screened, and had been for several years prior to 1990, and even though everyone at the hospital involved with the transfusion gave me much gentle reassurance, it was still a frightening prospect.

I went ahead with the massive transfusions.

According to Bruce, when the Spaulding doctors heard this news, although they received it calmly, their expressions changed completely.

"In that case," Dr. Stein said quietly, "we should go ahead with the test."

Since I was then relatively cognizant, I could, and did, consent to the test.

Three days of unbearable waiting for Bruce followed. He tried to put it out of his head by keeping busy, taking care of the children, and visiting me, hiding his concern. But I learned later that he was haunted by my fear about the transfusion—and how he had urged me to go through with it. I wasn't terribly worried, probably because I still couldn't process emotions and concerns the way I had before I got sick. However, I did momentarily recall the tennis player, Arthur Ashe, a sportsman I had always admired. I met him once at an exhibition tennis match at the old Detroit Tennis Club. As a painfully shy twelve-year-old, I mustered my courage to ask Ashe, then a rising star, for his autograph. A thorough gentleman, Ashe honored my request without hesitation and thrilled his young admirer. Years later, he died after contracting AIDS from tainted blood received during a transfusion following his heart surgery.

Bruce remembered another chilling thought: symptoms of the AIDS virus often took eight years or more to reveal themselves, and Westy's eighth birthday was just one month away.

Three days after the test, Bruce arrived at the hospital with the children. He found himself face-to-face in the elevator with Dr. Sandhu, who told him, "I have some news. There is a conference room on the eighth floor where we can talk."

He said nothing on the ride up. Bruce's heart was pounding.

"I was thinking about you," B.G. would tell me later. "I was thinking about Westy and Lindsay standing right there beside me. The memory of your decision to accept the transfusion still haunted me, because I had encouraged it, despite your concerns."

The elevator doors opened. Bruce and the children followed Dr. Sandhu down the hall to a bright conference room that overlooked the river. As soon as they were inside, Dr. Sandhu closed the door and turned to face Bruce.

"We have some very good news," he said. "The test came back negative."

◆ ◆ ◆

I quickly discovered that weekends at hospitals were tough, lonesome times. Though I know that it was hard for him to watch me struggle, Bruce always came, and often with the kids in tow, which brought me the greatest joy. Whenever B.G. appeared in my room, it felt like my whole world had arrived. But in general, there weren't nearly as many visitors as during the week, nor as many scheduled activities to keep one's mind off one's problems. There were different therapists and different nurses: no Teresa! But on my first weekend at Spaulding, I had my work cut out for me. The episode with my children, being unable to hug them and or mother them, left me feeling empty and sad. Then, while I was being fed some applesauce late one Friday afternoon, Hilly came to visit. At the same time, I had a little itch on the tip of my nose. To deal with it myself, I had to drop my head down to where my arms were. I had been sitting—propped up, actually—in the wheelchair.

"May I help?" Hilly asked.

"No, no," I said. "Thanks, I think I can do it."

What a ridiculous posture I was in. What a ridiculous situation, I thought. I saw the look of concern on Hilly's face that he tried unsuccessfully to conceal.

This just won't do, I thought to myself.

I was determined to solve the problem. I just didn't know how. The next day, a Saturday, there were no therapy sessions scheduled, no one to consult with, nor anyone to offer guidance. But I knew what needed to be done. I had to get my fingers to bend. I had an important first, private goal: I had to be able to caress my children's heads.

I also wanted to be a little less dependent in the event that I ever again had a tickle on the tip of my nose.

During that first weekend in the hospital, after my regular caregivers had gone off their shifts, I worked. I worked constantly to try to bend my fingers and lift my arms. But my insubordinate, leaden limbs would not respond to the signals that my brain—and my will—were sending them, quietly and furiously, without let up. I kept thinking and trying. I visualized the moment I would be able to do what I wanted. For hours and hours that turned into days,

I tried with all of my feeble might and persistent willpower to get my fingers to bend and to raise my arms. I worked as hard as I could before falling asleep. Then I woke up and began the process again. Over and over again.

It just has to happen, I thought. I must be able to do this.

It's so simple!

After hours and hours and days of work, things actually—miraculously—began to change. It began with the tips of my fingers. Starting with that small success, I slowly but gradually got my fingers to bend. Then my elbows. I honestly don't remember the exact sequence now, but I tried everything I could think of to get my fingers to bend and my arms to go up. Hour after hour, day after day, I tried. Then I fell asleep. Then I woke up and tried some more, again and again.

But from those first tiny successes, my body must have learned something, because gradually, things began to happen. Things began to somehow come together.

First thing Monday morning June 15, Teresa McLaughlin stepped into my room. She took one look and shrieked, "Oh, my God!"

On Friday, I had been a quadriplegic who could move only my neck. Now I was wiggling my fingers with my arms raised straight up in the air: *touchdown!* I didn't say a word. I just beamed.

"Get in here, come here!" Teresa called to everyone she could find in the corridor to witness what was obviously a bigger triumph than even I had realized. Returning to me Teresa said, "God love ya'," as she threw her arms around me in a celebratory hug.

Shortly after, I was able to do a squat-pivot transfer without the sliding board. This meant some strength was returning to my legs. I was thrilled to have graduated from the use of that particular item.

It was too early for anyone to truly know, but I was on my way toward leaving the hospital on my own steam.

◆ ◆ ◆

Physician's progress note

June 15, 1998

Estimated Length of Stay: Twelve weeks from admission; may reduce given dramatic improvement.

—P. Sandhu, MD

Physician's progress note

June 16, 1998

Patient in good spirits. Pleased with removal of trach. Still with considerable air leakage, though speech is clear ... Strength improving daily—now starting to get some return in her flexors.

—J. Stein, MD

At this time, the therapists also made casts of my lower legs and feet in order to prevent foot drop, which is weakness of the muscles that lift up the foot. This is often the first sign of muscular weakness from a number of neurological disorders. These weren't especially comfortable, but somehow, it seemed like progress.

The early days of my therapy at Spaulding also produced some welcome light moments. After my tracheostomy plug was removed, but before my throat had healed, I had a tendency to produce some dramatic and unusual sounds. This was due to air leakage, and the noises were completely unpredictable, uncontrollable, and loud.

"Honk," I would erupt, more or less spontaneously, usually in the middle of a therapy session. The weirdness and volume of the sound always took us by surprise. "Love me, love my pet goose," was all I could muster in the way of a rejoinder.

But any laughs at all were welcome, in that place, at that time.

Physician's progress note:

June 18, 1998

Blood pressure done today; [patient] feels tired, but asking to work on physical therapy. Virus [detected] today. Will watch for future signs of infection.

—C. Hay, MD

However surprising my early gains, my travails were not close to being over. Despite what was a dramatic beginning on the road to recovery, the doctors were still unwilling to paint an optimistic picture. Dr. Karen Furie, Spaulding's neurologist, took Bruce aside one day in mid-June to outline the possible scenarios.

"I think you should know that this progress might not continue," she said. "There are three possible outcomes. She could continue to improve. She could plateau, meaning her progress could end at any time. Or she could regress. We have to be cautiously pessimistic, and you should be prepared for whatever happens."

Physician's progress note:

June 19, 1998

Neurology: I have seen her daily, and she has been improving. Alert, fluent, oriented. Still some confusion about the timing of events. Confabulates about her daily routine … Had a long discussion with her mother and husband regarding her progress and plans for further Rx [rehabilitation or acute care therapy] if she plateaus or deteriorates.

—K. Furie, MD

Bruce did not want to burden himself with speculation. He did not want to look into the future for fear of what the future might bring.

I disciplined myself to not ask questions. There was so little data on the disorder that looking ahead, even to the next day, didn't seem worthwhile.

—Bruce

Apparently, the doctors felt the same way.

When we know the natural history of a disorder, we have a pretty good sense of how patients are going to do. But in Wendy's case, we still didn't know what had caused her condition. We took things day by day and tried not to over-prognosticate.

—J. Stein, MD

♦ ♦ ♦

B.G. wrote a heart-rending note after I had begun to show progress.

My Dear,

Now that you are thankfully regaining your strength, you should know that when your condition was deteriorating, I cried for three days. I looked around our home and realized that it was all yours—the style, the art, even the kids. The kids and I have just been lucky to enjoy it. I suddenly felt very small ...

—B.G.

It broke my heart to think that B.G. could ever have felt small. He had been so magnificent, in so many ways, throughout our ordeal.

♦ ♦ ♦

My second weekend at Spaulding was unusually discouraging. I had an alternate physical therapist, whose name I conveniently forgot. He probably wasn't a bad fellow, but he inadvertently told me something that shattered my morale.

Ever the researcher, I brought up the subject of myelin with him.[5] To put it diplomatically, the young therapist did not properly filter the information he relayed to me. "The rate at which the myelin sheath returns, on a linear basis," he began, "is extremely slow—miniscule, actually. It's a minute fraction of an inch per month—if it occurs at all."

"Are you sure about this?" I pleaded, and not a little bit stunned. "Things have already begun to happen, you know."

Only toward the end of our session did he touch upon the unpredictable nature of re-myelination and address the myelin sheath's potential to return in "pockets," rather than in a linear progression.

This was a conversation that demonstrated what havoc a little knowledge could wreak. It was a real spirit killer.

♦ ♦ ♦

In a continuation of the research begun at Beth Israel-Deaconess, tests were done nearly every day at Spaulding in the ongoing effort to determine the cause of my disorder. Pages upon pages of test results were returned, nearly all of them negative. On balance, this was more good news than bad. While the results did not illuminate the origins of my neurological mishap, so many negative outcomes pointed to it being mono-phasal, meaning a one-time event.

There continued to be an abundance of theories regarding my disorder. Dr. Furie thought it could have been something as simple as a sinus infection gone haywire near the brain. Coincident to that idea, early in my stay at Spaulding, I was awakened for a midnight procedure by one of the duty nurses who I hadn't seen before. She was taken aback.

"What are you doing on a stroke floor?" she asked. She was young, wiry, and bespectacled. "So young. What happened to you?"

We fell into conversation and quickly discovered that we shared an enthusiasm for gardening.

"When you work in the garden," she asked, "do you wear all the protective gear? Boots? Gloves?"

"Yes ... yes," I answered.

"A mask?"

"A mask?" I echoed.

"A mask. You should always wear a mask when you garden ... And do you have any wild animals in your yard?"

"Animals come through our yard most every night," I said. "Possum, raccoon, even resident skunks from time to time."

My answers were becoming more interesting to her.

"Where do they come from?" was her next question. "Don't you live right *in* town?"

"It's been a bad year for skunks, in town," I explained. "But we also live near a 4,500-acre wildlife refuge.

"You should always wear a mask when you garden," she repeated. "You never know what bacteria the animals coming through your yard could be depositing from dander or feces. If the bacteria become airborne, things can get complicated."

This was a conversation I didn't forget. A story recounted to me just a few days later paralleled the nurse's information.

An old friend, Mary Stone, called from Darien, Connecticut. "We have a neighbor who had a sickness just like yours," said Mary. "He had been working in his yard before he was stricken. It was traced to bacteria left by rodents scrambling around his woodpile."

I thought back to May 10, 1998, which was Mother's Day. Bruce and the kids took me down to Longhill, the old Sedgewick estate in Beverly, Massachusetts. It served as the headquarters of the Trustees of Reservations, the oldest conservation organization in the country. Each Mother's Day, the trustees held a rare plant auction and sale, which I enjoyed, and Westy and Lindsay loved to ride around the old estate in the hay wagons. Visiting Longhill was better than any expensive brunch at a crowded restaurant or country club.

The weather could not have been worse that day. It poured buckets of rain, the wind howled, and it was bone-chilling cold. I got my plants, though. Soaked and cold, we piled back in the car so that crazy mom could return to her garden. I put in a few plants, but the wind was blowing so hard off the harbor from the northeast that I was afraid the blossoms would be damaged. I placed the rest of my purchases on our patio out back, in the lee of the house, and puttered elsewhere around the yard. I wore long pants, boots, gloves, and a slicker—but no mask. And just for something to do outside, I rearranged the woodpile.

In the early days of my stay at Beth Israel-Deaconess, Dr. Zaleznik, the infectious disease specialist, had noted that I had been working avidly in the garden before falling ill. Might it have been fatal?

♦ ♦ ♦

Despite my somewhat loopy cheerfulness, there were definite frustrations. My will was firmly in place, but little else. I knew what I had to do. However, possessing the strength to do it was a matter over which I had little control.

In his progress notes for June 17, Dr. Stein had written, "rapid neurological recovery continues." Though my mind was bouncing back, it was a different story with my body. I remained as weak and impaired as one could imagine. For an entire week at the beginning of my demanding physical therapy, my blood pressure dropped precipitously during the workouts. This left me dizzy, lightheaded, and feeling weaker than ever.

"How can I possibly get back the strength to do the work I know I need to do?" I wondered, almost in desperation.

Strength was crucial. But my impairment, weight loss, and the long time spent in bed resulted in muscle atrophy. All of these worked against my regaining strength.

Dr. Stein responded. To combat my orthostatic hypotension (the medical phrase for the drop in blood pressure that results from suddenly sitting up or standing up) he ordered both intravenous saline and salt tablets four times daily. The improvement in my stamina was apparent within days. I finally felt that I could apply myself to the work at hand.

What I didn't realize, however, was that I still needed a miracle.

Physician's progress note:

June 22, 1998

[Patient] had dramatic improvement in upper extremities and lower extremities strength this last week ... Trach was pulled on June 16

... Patient encouraged to eat more ... Estimated length of stay: eight weeks from now; may reduce given dramatic improvement.

—P. Sandhu, MD

Other stumbling blocks were a lack of food and sleep. Although my trach was gone, a feeding tube remained. This allowed me to graduate to regular, but soft, food (such as pureed vegetables). My nurses and therapists worked to teach me "propulsion swallowing," a method of vigorously moving the food down to my stomach. The goal was to remove my feeding tube, but this could not happen until I could take in sufficient amounts of nutrition on my own.

Dr. Stein was disappointed with my caloric intake. "You're eating enough for a large bird, perhaps," he gently scolded one day, "but not for a grown woman."

I had never been a big eater. But with the help of calorie boosters such as Jevity and Ensure, liquids administered through the PEG tube directly into my stomach, I did begin to beef up a bit. That, coupled with a decent night's sleep, allowed me to begin in earnest the most difficult physical task I had ever undertaken. Learning to walk again was a task I ranked right up with childbirth, which came in second because it didn't take as long.

I undertook numerous exercises to strengthen my trunk so I could sit without flopping. My hips were weak and uncontrollable. The muscles around my knees had a tendency to buckle or lock. After raising my arms that first weekend at Spaulding, I set a second, private, goal to draw my knees up in bed. This seemed within the realm of possibility, but it took nearly a week to accomplish. I was trying so hard to move everything I could—and things I couldn't. Once again, my limbs felt as if they were made of lead. I would draw up my feet a few inches in the bed, and then, ever so slowly, my knees would follow. My modus operandi was to exercise anything I could move, if only my toes.

"If these little victories keep coming, they might add up to something," I explained to B.G. "Besides, I have plenty of time for practice."

Through all of this, Westy and Lindsay were my great motivation. When I was in the intensive care unit at Beth Israel-Deaconess, Bruce brought in a framed photograph of the children taken on the beach at Plum Island for our last Christmas card. Of course, the picture accompanied me to Spaulding. Whenever I looked at that beautiful photograph and saw their sweet faces peering up at me, it made me work harder than I once might have thought possible. More than anything, I wanted to be Mom again, and I wanted to be whole. Although I knew it could be done, I wanted to be a mom without a wheelchair, the mom I'd been. I wanted to be the one who, as Westy always said when I did something he really liked, earned a "WowMom."

I *had* to succeed for those beautiful kids of mine. When the leaden weight of my legs seemed overwhelming, I looked at the picture, and that was all it took to spur me on. I made a little more progress each day, and I do mean little, no more than a couple of inches a day, and on some days, perhaps no more than a half inch.

I remember thinking, "I just have to be able to get those knees up. If I can clear this one hurdle, if I can just do it, I'll be one step closer to walking out of here."

This was an important, private milestone. Again, I struggled for days, hour after hour in my bed between therapy sessions.

About a week after I'd begun this particular campaign, it finally happened. "Look what I can do!" I said to Teresa in triumph one morning as I drew up my knees. She shook her head in disbelief.

My progress continued. What other people remembered most from that time at Spaulding was my absolute determination to walk out of that place.

I was demented in my determination. My therapists recall bizarre scenes that I exorcised from my memory bank. One day early on, for example, I was brought back to my room, and the therapists began to explain how they would help me back into bed.

"Oh, that's okay," I chirped, trying to save them their trouble. "I'll just hop in by myself. I'll be fine." As I flopped in my wheelchair, continuing to stay exactly where I was, the therapists exchanged looks of concerned disbelief at my profound lack of self-awareness.

On another occasion, the therapists tried with no success to get me to perform some sort of minimal movement. As they tried to move me onto the next therapeutic experiment, I became insubordinate.

"Wait, I think I can do that," I said. "Just give me another minute."

Then I lay there, staring up at the ceiling, gritting my teeth, as nothing moved. No matter how hard I squeezed my inner core of will, nothing moved; nothing happened. I could hardly believe it. I didn't understand why nothing was happening. But I kept trying. The willfulness was there in spades. The therapists gently humored me. But as hard as I tried, as much as I desired to have my body working again, nothing much happened in those first days and weeks.

The therapists had to steer me along, however, and after ten or fifteen minutes of watching the sheer failure of my willpower, they got me to acquiesce by speaking as one would to a willful toddler. "We'll help you just this once," was the gentle line with which they bribed me in order to keep the process moving.

♦ ♦ ♦

What was happening with my children during the time their mother was absent?

When I read my medical record in detail several months later, the single most jarring entry was the note from Dr. Dori Zaleznik, the infectious disease chief at Beth Israel-Deaconess. Her medical note for May 20, my first full day at Beth Israel-Deaconess and two days before I became deeply comatose, indicated I was unaware of my children: "Unable to say where she lives or if she has children." Now, more than one month later, as I continued the most difficult physical work I will probably ever face, it would be those forgotten children who would give me the ultimate motivation I needed.

Bruce was magnificent as he dealt on a daily basis with the medical horror in Boston. He spent time meeting with doctors, researching, and advocating—then returning home and putting on a smile for Westy and Lindsay.

The overwhelming sense in my early days at Beth Israel-Deaconess was that I wouldn't make it. This was an awful time for Bruce as he prepared, in the worst-case scenario, to tell our children that their mother had died. Bruce managed their care throughout this time. By all accounts, Westy and Lindsay came through the ordeal intact. The children understood that I was sick in the hospital and the doctors were working hard to help me get better. It was an extraordinary balancing act on Bruce's part. As my mother later said of Bruce, "He did everything possible to see that the children did things in as normal a way as possible."

Other relatives, friends, and nannies also stepped into the breach. The psychologist at Westy's school was on deck, in case her services were needed. Neighbors and acquaintances, including some I hardly knew, baked and cooked and brought food to the house. Gabriele Atkinson, a friend and former nanny, filled our home with flowers and took Westy to the movies. The Eblings entertained everyone from Grandma Billie to Lindsay. These were the greatest gifts, knowing that my children were happily distracted and otherwise occupied.

June 21 was Father's Day. Friends brought in cards for the children and me to give to Bruce. Everything I had been able to do before the onset of my illness had been profoundly diminished, including that of being able to hold a pen and write. I pressed the button to raise my bed, and, with difficulty, got hold of a pen. Then I struggled to write a sentiment to B.G. for his special day.

It took me a long time to write it because I had so little control. And it was difficult for him to decipher. But my message came across. He looked at it and moved on rather quickly, but I later learned that it was a tough moment for him.

> *June 26. 1998*
>
> My dearest darling,
>
> I ~~don't~~ know what I would have done without you these last week. My darling, I love you so much. YOU HAVE DONE SO MUCH — more than anyone else could have done for me! Honey, I will never forget all what you have done. [illegible lines] will fill me everything, saving me from ????.
>
> I love you so much, dearest, dearest darling.
>
> Love, Me

I was moved to see that you had written something that was obviously so difficult for you, and I remember feeling relieved that you were able to write it at all. But it was greatly different from how you were before.

I thought it might be the best you would ever be able to do—and that I would take care of you for the rest of your life.

—Bruce

Both children, I sensed, were somewhat intimidated by the hospital. It was an environment different than any they had ever experienced, and I was right in the middle of it all, not looking or acting quite like myself. That was where their mom lived now; where she slept. They were much more familiar with the sight of their mom racing up and down three flights of stairs, literally running a household. Now she was flat on her back, unable to move anything very well except her neck and head. Scores of people they didn't know hovered about her, waiting on her hand and foot, and clinicians doing their work. Their "WowMom" had become a memory.

I began to believe that at some level I had lost Lindsay—lost her trust. I would have to work hard to win her back. As loopy as I was, when she began to visit me, I distinctly sensed a distance between us. It could have been puzzlement or worse. She was not quite three and one-half years old when I fell ill, and she couldn't see me for four weeks. The separation was completely unexpected; there had been no time to prepare her. When she did see me, I was flat on my back, unable to move even to hug her, and hooked up to IV lines and an artificial breathing apparatus.

I had often read a favorite bedtime story to her that was about a family of owlets who worry when mother owl goes off at night to hunt. In the story, of course, the owl mommy always returned. In an effort to assuage the separation anxiety that reared up in Lindsay from time to time, I would read the book and say, "Now, see? What do mommies always do? They always come back!"

When I, lying flat on my back at Spaulding, recalled this ritual, I could only think, *My God, what have I done? She'll never believe me again.*

One could only guess at what went on in the mind of my young daughter. Given Lindsay's presumed inability to understand something as complex as her mother's long absence, even for a logical reason, I was concerned that she might feel rejected. I believed that I would have to mount a campaign to win her back. I had Bruce put her on the phone as often as possible. He was diligent about making extra drives down from the North Shore with the children, not always an easy thing to do. How many French fries and chicken nuggets Lindsay winged from her car seat will never be known. How many overturned milkshakes?

"I love you, Button," I said each time I had Lindsay's ear. "Do you know that I think about you *all the time?*"

Will she ever be close to me again? I wondered as I lay in my hospital bed. *Will she ever trust me? Be my friend? Will I ever be able to care for her again? Will I be able to hold my children in my arms? Nurse them when they're sick?*

Some of Lindsay's wide-eyed questions broke my heart.

"Are you coming home today, Mommy?" she once asked, as she sat on the foot of my hospital bed.

"I would *love* to come home with you today, but the doctors won't let me," was the only answer I could give. "They still have a lot of work to do to make me all better."

The disappointment in her downcast eyes was obvious. Yet she also seemed to accept the situation with a degree of grace that amazed me in a child so young. At some level, she must have understood my limitations.

I vaguely remember that during my early days at Spaulding, friends from my office had come to visit. Bruce and Lindsay were there, too. We were in the solarium, down the hall from my room. The day was warm, and the sun, reflecting on the river, beat in the windows. I was in my wheelchair, pretty much flopped over, as usual, barely able to sit up, and Lindsay had just been put on my lap.

I tried very hard to put my arms around her, but I just couldn't do it. Apparently Lindsay didn't even want me to touch her that day.

"No, Mommy," she said as I tried. "Don't touch me. You're sick!"

At nearly eight years old, Westy was capable of greater understanding. One evening at Spaulding during his visit, he seemed rather quiet.

"Honey," I said, "are you okay?"

"Yes, Mom."

"Do you like coming to the hospital?" I asked.

"Yes, I do, Mom."

"What do you like best about the hospital?"

"Seeing you."

That little statement, spoken so quietly, was the best thing I could have heard. Regardless of my doubts and worries about my much younger Lindsay, and despite the long time away, there was no question about Westy being firmly in my fold.

◆ ◆ ◆

On my third weekend at Spaulding, I had an opportunity to return a semblance of normalcy into my children's lives.

"Why don't you get out as a family and get away from the hospital?" Dr. Stein suggested. "A lot of people like to visit the Science Museum nearby, but you can go off anywhere you want, for a few hours."

That Saturday, which was June 20, Bruce drove in early to get a lesson from Dawn, my primary therapist, on how to transfer me between our car and my wheelchair. (B.G. could figure out how to do anything, but the lesson was required!) As Westy and Lindsay watched closely with anticipation to see what I could do, we practiced this operation a few times. Once we passed muster, we won our ticket out.

It was the nicest day, by far, in a month of record-setting rainfall. We decided to go to the Boston Public Garden, a long overdue visit. Westy hadn't been on the swan boats since he was two, and Lindsay had never been on them. The children were especially happy that day.

It was exciting for us to do something fun together as a family once again, for B.G. and me to be able to do something nice for the kids—and away from the hospital, just like old times. After all the rain, the weather was perfect. It was especially wonderful for us all to be outdoors. In my cloistered hospital environment, I had forgotten so many everyday sensations like the scents of the outdoors—not just the flowers, but the evergreens and the grass as well. That day, every sensation seemed so rich. The children played on the inviting sculpture of Mrs. Mallard and her ducklings, and the concessionaires who ran the Swan Boats could not have been more accommodating.

They even understood the language of physical therapy. "Would you like to transfer to the boat seat or go in your wheelchair?" they asked. "We'll do whatever you want."

Once I realized that it was possible for me to sit in a regular seat, I thought it would be encouraging for the kids to see me out of my wheelchair and looking more like their old mom—even though I was far from being able to walk.

We had a boat almost entirely to ourselves, so there we were, looking like any all-American family enjoying a trip on the Swan Boats in the Public Garden. The difference, of course, was the wheelchair waiting for me back at the dock.

It was a convincing show. Afterward, as Bruce and Westy took turns pushing me through the Garden, Lindsay, who sat on my lap for most of the outing, continually looked at me, saucer-eyed, repeating her earnest little question, "Mommy, are you all better?"

♦ ♦ ♦

Bruce brought the children in one morning on their way to Cape Cod to visit his family. I was elated to see them, as usual, and Westy and Lindsay were excited at the prospect of soon being on the beach with their cousins. Before they left the hospital, the three of them accompanied me to the gym for a physical therapy session with Dawn. Bruce had observed many therapy sessions, but the kids had not, because he wanted to shield them from having to see me struggle too much. But we all had a sense that this one would be different.

As she put me through my routine strengthening exercises, she had a sudden suggestion, "Let's try something different," Dawn said impulsively. She brought out a tall, four-wheel, bilateral, forearm support vehicle known as an Atlas Walker, which was used to help people re-learn to walk.

She and two assistant therapists wheeled me to the oddly imposing contraption and locked my wheelchair in place. Then they hoisted me into position, a task more easily described than done. Raising my dead weight, even with three people helping, was exhausting work. But once my arms were resting on the high support and my feeble, useless legs were leaning against the lower support, I was able to wheel myself—able to *walk* in a way—a few feet down the hall. While I wasn't actually walking of my own accord, it was exciting. And arduous—I became light-headed after moving forward just a few feet.

But for me, it was exhilarating, and for Bruce and the kids, it was a wonderful sight.

After my family left, I thanked Dawn, "That was a real morale booster."

"I knew it would be," she said, as she looked down at me with a knowing little smile.

◆ ◆ ◆

"I was amazed that by June 24, you were walking fifteen feet with the Atlas Walker," Dawn would tell me. "That was significant, and from there, you just continued to go." But it was not until the end of June, during one of Foster's visits, did I have the nerve to articulate my goal of walking unaided out of Spaulding, with my family. At that point, there was still a tremendous amount of hard work ahead of me and much uncertainty. Still, the goal remained paramount.

"I don't want any of the paraphernalia, you know," I told my dear friend, struggling to maintain my composure as I focused on the picture of Westy and Lindsay. "I want to *walk* out of here, with my family."

Foster listened intently, then after only a moment's hesitation, said, "I have no doubt that you will."

As I became more adept at moving around in my wheelchair and the weather improved, I ventured outside more often. My usual destinations were the hospital patio or the pier, down on the Charles River, to exercise whatever was moving. I always thought of Spaulding's riverside location as such a gift. With the arrival of summer, I suggested to my young occupational therapy aide, Kate Schaefer, that we work outside. Kate came every afternoon with a dowel, weights, and thera-putty, a thick, clay-like substance, which she used to help strengthen the muscles in my hands.

The fresh air, sunshine, and breezes off the Charles were so wonderful and uplifting that I almost forgot I was supposed to be in Maine. I sat outside with friends and family who came to visit—the children loved to feed the ducks and pigeons, and B.G. always preferred to be outdoors. I also visited with other patients outdoors. Even though I couldn't walk, it felt good to be able to move around independently in my wheelchair. At that point, I could get to therapy sessions on my own instead of being picked up and brought back to my room. Yet I never did become terribly adept at operating the chair. The lack of skill was possibly a manifestation of a secret rebellion: I didn't want a wheelchair in my life.

Several patients on my floor became my new old friends. Some told me they had monitored my progress from the day I arrived.

Sally Frank was the wife of my courtly next-door neighbor, Dr. Howard Frank, a renowned cardiologist at Beth Israel-Deaconess who had suffered a debilitating stroke the month before I was felled. Sally visited her husband every day. "I remember," she told me, "when you first came in. I thought how awful it was for such a young person to be so sick."

Sometimes, I stopped to visit with Dr. Frank.

One Sunday morning, I found him waiting outside his room in his wheelchair, alone in the corridor, and I stopped to say hello. He turned to me, took my hand, and said carefully, "I feel a little low."

I felt so helpless and hoped so much that Sally, his brother, Edward, or another of his frequent visitors, would soon walk down the hall. "I am sure Sally will be here any minute," I said. "You know she comes every day, and she always looks so nice for you." This was the only thing I could think of for him to hold onto.

Just then, with perfect timing, Sally, Edward, and Edward's daughter did come walking down the hall. "Look, Dr. Frank," I said, relieved. "They're all here."

"I think I am going to weep," said the kindly old prince as I left him in the comfort of his family.

Bert and Sterra Takeff also became new friends from down the hall. Bert had suffered a stroke. Sterra, another lovely and engaging wife, visited her husband every day. Indeed, toward the end of my stay, the fourth floor at Spaulding Hospital reminded me a bit of college dorm life—visiting buddies down the hall and being delighted by visits in return. Time and again, these brief episodes pointed to the most important part of life: the people we love, the people we can care for, even in a small way and if only for a short time. In the rush to prioritize our lives, nothing else comes close.

♦ ♦ ♦

"B.G., you must go to Vermont as we planned," I said to my wonderful husband. "You can't do any more here, and you'll have a great time. It'll be good for you to get away."

I was insisting that Bruce, who seemed a bit hesitant to leave me, carry on with our plans to take the children and join our great friends, Leslie Sennott and Bill Johnston, with their children, in Vermont. Leslie and I had made these plans during the winter. Their son, Tucker, and Westy would go to a sleep-away camp for the first time, at the Merck Forest. The adults and the little girls, Lindsay, Katharine, and Victoria, would relax at the charming old farmhouse in the mountains above Dorset that Bruce and I had used as a ski-house for more than twenty years. He would be able to enjoy a few days with good friends, and the children would have fun in a beautiful setting. It would be a distracting and much-needed respite for them. I had hoped that it would allow them to conjure different thoughts from those their many visits to the hospital brought up: whether they would ever see their wife and mother walking again. The doctors were encouraged, but still did not know how far I would progress.

I had called Leslie to let her know how strongly I wanted them all to stick to our plans of long ago. "It's not as though you're taking Bruce away," I stated. "There's nothing more he can do here now. It'll be good for him. I *insist* that you go."

However, a new problem was developing. For several days, I had been waking up with sharp pains on the right side of my head—the side where the lesions had been discovered. I tried not to wander down that path very far.

Bruce and the children left for their little vacation with the Johnstons in Vermont on June 24.

Physician's progress notes:

June 23, 1998

Neurology:

Ms. Ford complains of right temporal headache two or three days in a row, associated with nasal congestion and mild nausea. No visual symptoms. Fully oriented. Able to do serial 7s (multiplication of 7), name her watch, crystal, and band. Follows complex commands. Stammered over words several times. I am concerned that she has recurrence of the symptoms that heralded her illness. Neurologically, there has been no decline. Reconsider lumbar puncture: this might provide early evidence of relapse and be an indication for further diagnostic/therapeutic interventions.

—K. Furie, MD

Physician's progress notes:

June 24, 1998

Patient continues to improve … Able to walk a few steps yesterday in Physical Therapy … Still mild headaches, but improving … Eating well on soft diet.

—J. Stein, MD

Whenever I woke up with a headache, I called for the nurses, who promptly gave me intravenous Tylenol. The medication never failed to alleviate the pain, and rather quickly, so I had no complaints. But the headaches inevitably returned the following morning, strong pains of the sort I had never before experienced.

As the headaches continued, Dr. Karen Furie, Spaulding's neurologist, came to speak with me. "There may be another lumbar puncture in your future," she said sympathetically. "We do not anticipate a problem, but based on your history, we feel we should be cautious."

I'd had two spinal taps already, one at the local hospital on the North Shore at the beginning of this awful medical adventure, the second at Beth Israel-Deaconess. I remembered neither.

"I've had two babies and epidurals with each delivery," I told Dr. Furie. "A spinal tap can't be much worse. If something is wrong, we should know."

Physician's progress notes:

June 25, 1998

Attending:

Patient still with headaches, but no other symptoms. Discussed with Dr. Furie—repeat lumbar puncture planned ... Consider repeat MRI based on lumbar puncture results.

—J. Stein, MD

Neurology:

Patient awoke again with right temporal headache—seems more severe. [No] associated neurological deficits have developed. Still improving functionally. In light of her persistent symptoms, I explained risks and benefits of lumbar puncture, and she consented to the procedure ... Approximately 12 cc of clear CSF (cerebral spinal fluid) was obtained. There were no complications ... Discussed CSF studies with infectious diseases ...

—K. Furie, MD

Dr. Furie remained in close contact with Dr. Scammell at Beth Israel-Deaconess. Together, they formulated a plan that—depending on what the lumbar puncture revealed—could have meant my return to Beth Israel-Deaconess for another MRI. I did not wish to burden my husband with this possibility.

"I told Dr. Stein that you wanted to keep this from Bruce," Teresa McLaughlin confessed one morning around that time. "I hope you don't mind. I was concerned that he might be on the phone with Bruce, as he often is, and spill the beans."

Dr. Stein knew I was fully cognizant and that my wishes had to be respected, but he still thought Bruce should know. The day before the lumbar puncture was scheduled, Dr. Stein and Dr. Sandhu sought me out in the gym, in the middle of a therapy session.

"I know you're trying to keep the test from Bruce," Dr. Stein said. "I'd just like to say that if it were my wife going through this, I would want to know."

I remained adamant. Knowing that my family was having a good time with great friends in a beautiful place, away from the sadness and uncertainties of the hospital, made me very happy. I could not bring myself to worry them or disrupt their little holiday.

"I just can't do it," I told Dr. Stein, as I struggled through my exercises. "B.G. needs this time away from everything. The kids need it. And I don't want to spoil things for them up there."

The morning of the procedure, I awakened with the worst headache of this entire period. At lunchtime, I had a number of visitors and asked a pal from my office if she would stay, thinking it might help if I had a familiar hand to squeeze. Teresa also was there, as well as my team of therapists, four of them, who had never seen a spinal tap done before. Finally, Dr. Gruzyna Piskorska, a kidney specialist who had been called in for consultation, arrived just as Dr. Furie started the procedure.

The spinal tap was done in my room. Dr. Furie was calm and reassuring. Women who have borne children usually have had experience with needles in the spine, and to me, this was no different. Lying in the fetal position, as directed, I couldn't even see the three-inch-long needle, which was probably all to the good. The procedure actually did not hurt that much. Dr. Furie gave me extra anesthesia, and with all those supportive women surrounding me, the medical theatre going on in my room was actually rather comforting.

Tim Hollingworth showed up that evening for a visit and found me flat on my back, per doctor's orders, to avoid strong headaches that could ensue from the procedure. I swore him to secrecy before explaining what had happened and why I couldn't sit up.

"You can't tell *anyone*," I remember emphasizing to him. People had worried enough.

Several days later, we learned the spinal fluid was normal and that there would be no need for a return to Beth Israel-Deaconess and additional MRIs. Ironically, the day after the procedure, the early-morning headaches began to abate.

I thought I detected a collective sigh of relief, but I did not learn until much later the true depth of concern about a recurrence of ADEM. This little episode in my recovery process was more than a minor blip. Dr. Furie's calm manner belied a real worry that was shared by my fourth-floor medical team.

"We hadn't seen any physical changes," Dawn would tell me, "but people wondered if there were other things going on, besides the headaches."

◆ ◆ ◆

That evening, I was about to drift off to sleep when a new doctor walked into my room. Arnold Shaw, a courtly, young infectious disease specialist from

Massachusetts General, had come by to introduce himself. He was especially interested in my situation. I discerned a real curiosity and decided to tell him everything I could remember that might bear on my case. "Who knows?" I thought. "This might be the person who discovers the cause of this whole adventure."

He listened to my story, and I learned quite a bit from him as well. He went out of his way to get a sneak preview from the lab of my spinal tap results. He was able to report that there was a reassuringly low level of white blood cells. A high count could have indicated the possibility of a recurrence of ADEM. He also explained the operations of the National Centers for Disease Control in Atlanta, which had been sent a number of my serums for analysis, the formidable resources in Boston having been exhausted.

"It might be years before they determine what caused your illness," as Dr. Shaw summed up, "or, it might never be resolved."

◆ ◆ ◆

The nurses agreed that I had one distinct area of weakness: shots. I promised the phlebotomists, who drew my blood, that I wouldn't scream. But I did have to vent in some way. Usually, it was, "*OHGODOHGODOHGODGOD"* in as low a voice as I could manage. I had plenty of practice. To prevent blood clots in my legs that could result from being almost constantly bedridden, shots of Heparin were administered into my stomach twice each day, once in the early morning and again at bedtime. Six weeks times seven days a week, times two shots a day equaled eighty-four shots just to my stomach alone. After a while, the nurses actually had difficulty finding a place that wasn't bruised.

"Inhale deeply now," Imelda Toleran, my favorite late-shift nurse, would advise. It must have been just enough of a distraction to minimize the pain, for she was one of the most adept at this particular task. There were a couple of other nurses who, for some reason, were also fairly successful at administering shots quickly and less painfully.

I was also party to an endless number of blood draws for sampling. Rarely a day passed that blood wasn't drawn for some sort of test, often before I had finished breakfast. My blood was difficult to find. Plus, I had lost so much weight that my veins were hard and they often collapsed before a sufficient sample could be drawn. This typically resulted in another attempt, often to no avail.

"Don't worry," they promised, "we give up after three tries."

But the phlebotomists always came back. Many times they resorted to putting their needles into my thin, small hands because that was the only place they could see veins that seemed strong enough to withstand the punctures.

I felt like a human pincushion.

Early one afternoon, two nurses, Emily and Pat, appeared at my door to insert a catheter into my left arm. The idea was to provide the needles a port for easier access. What transpired was nearly an hour of sheer physical torture. It was similar to the unsuccessful attempts to draw blood, but without letup. The procedure was further intensified due to the large needles and catheters being used and the complete absence of anesthesia.

The first attempt, which seemed to last forever, was unsuccessful. I could hardly believe it. "My God," I thought, "they have to do it again."

"Maybe we should give up," Emily quietly suggested to Pat. "Look at her. I don't know if I can stand this," I overheard Pat respond.

I asked the nurses if they had enough equipment to try again. When I learned that they did, I told them to try once more.

"Just go ahead and try to get it done—please," I said. I turned my head away and steeled myself as best I could. "We've come this far. I don't want to have to start all over again another time."

I did not look at the site. I just gritted my teeth and gripped the bed rails till my knuckles went white. I never screamed. I don't think I had the strength left over to scream.

The nurses were grateful that I allowed them to follow through. Ultimately, the procedure was successful.

A situation such as that must be a paradox for a nurse. To enter a profession because you are devoted to caring for people and want to help them and then to find yourself the instrument of such extraordinary pain must be difficult to reconcile.

Once the procedure was completed and I had caught my breath, Dr. Stein appeared. Dr. Stein was a great guy, but because he'd missed the big show, he had no idea how rough it had been. From my right arm, he proceeded to draw several vials of blood himself, and quite skillfully, causing minimal pain.

"Now," he said, in his pleasant way as he washed up, "that wasn't so bad, was it?"

I found this to be incredulous. I had difficulty finding the right words to describe what I had just endured. Because my cognitive ability was not back to normal and word retrieval was a problem, I couldn't come up with the right form of the word when it did finally come to me.

"The word I would use," I explained to Dr. Stein, "has something to do with barbarism."

◆ ◆ ◆

Sleep presented its own set of ongoing challenges. It was not possible to have an uninterrupted night's sleep in the hospital. Various procedures had to be done every four to six hours, and medications needed to be administered.

Also, my series of roommates had a tendency to talk out loud in the midnight hours. Some spoke in their native, and foreign, languages. This made their monologues even more disconcerting. I didn't understand them and, therefore, couldn't even learn anything from these late-night sessions. One roommate watched television constantly, which was difficult for me because it was not my habit at all. I often suspected that I could have been quite content living in the relative quiet of the mostly non-electronic nineteenth century.

Sleep was elusive. The morning weigh-in was one of only many reasons for an early wake-up call. The first time I was weighed, it was 5:00 AM. Two nurses brought in a portable scale. The contraption consisted of a canvas sling suspended from metal hoops.

"Does this really have to be done now?" I mumbled sleepily.

Apparently it did. Because it had to be done before breakfast, the task fell to the night nurses shortly before their shift ended. Still, it was one heck of a way to wake up. Fortunately, and for reasons I didn't understand, they never did it at the end of a night-shift again.

The other ongoing difficulty of my hospital life was the waiting. Waiting for food. Waiting to be bathed. Waiting for my nightly medications so that I would be free to fall asleep early. Waiting, hoping for visitors or phone calls. However, I do believe that medical staffers, over-scheduled and overworked virtually without exception, were as responsive as they could be. After they learned my preferences, they often anticipated them and delivered on them even before I made a request.

"Where else would I ever be taken to the shower with a pile of fresh towels on my lap?" I said to Teresa one day. "Where else would I be brought three meals a day on a tray in bed? And have mail and flowers delivered almost daily?"

The Spaulding Spa.

◆ ◆ ◆

By the time Dr. Sandu moved on to his next rotation at the end of June, my progress was swift and sometimes miraculously dramatic. I found that activities and exercises that were difficult on Monday became easier by Tuesday or Wednesday. New developments came faster and more furiously by the day.

After each little victory, I made phone calls to my tribe. Typically, this was Mom, Kim and Anne in Santa Fe, the Eblings, Elizabeth and her husband Bill in Michigan, Foster and Tim, and, of course, B.G., on the very few days that he wasn't in Boston with me and usually with the children in tow.

The last week in June, we held off on walking training and focused on strengthening your hip and pelvic musculature. This was a time for high-kneeling exercises and for exercising your quadrupeds, hands, and knees. Then we had you kneeling with various combinations of arm lifts.

Within the next week, the first week in July, we went from your Atlas Walker to a regular, handheld walker, to a straight cane. Then we got you on the stairs.

—Dawn Lucier

In the midst of my arduous struggle to walk again, I delivered a Knute Rockne speech of my own, to Dawn. I wanted to let her know how important she was to me. In Dawn, I had met my rehab match. Her diligence and perfectionism were exactly what I required. If she would give me her best—of which I had no doubt—I would certainly give her mine.

"You are now the most important person to me here," I told her. "You are the one person who can get me to walk again and can help me win back my life."

"I've always given it my all," Dawn replied, reflecting on her general approach to physical therapy. "I never give up, regardless of the hopelessness. I pretty much tax people to their physical limits."

In fact, I was so determined that I became an exercise outlaw. There were movements and activities that Dawn specifically warned me not to do in my room without a therapist, for fear that I would fall. The Spaulding staff was conscientious and extremely conservative about doing all in its power to prevent tumbles. A patient's lack of insight into his or her abilities was a common problem at rehab hospitals. Patients often thought they could walk when they couldn't. They believed they could function the way they remembered.

The high-kneeling exercise, in particular, was excruciatingly arduous. I was directed to kneel on a raised mat that was a couple of feet off the floor. This was an accomplishment in itself. I could barely raise myself without becoming lightheaded. For support, I rested my arms on a large plastic ball placed directly in front of me. Next, I lowered my trunk to a near-sitting position and, straightening my thighs again, raised myself back to the kneeling position. This may sound simple, but at the beginning, I nearly fainted each time I attempted it. I had lost so much weight and had suffered from muscle atrophy. What little musculature I retained wasn't functioning very well. Essentially, I had to hoist 115 pounds of dead weight. Often, I concentrated so intently on the work at hand that I had a tendency to hold my breath.

"Remember to breathe," the therapists reminded me, constantly. "Breathe!"

My light-headed feelings continued. Because the exercise seemed so minimal, I found it difficult to accept that I was having a hard time of it.

I caught myself remembering my competitive tennis days. "Tennis," I thought wistfully. "How will I ever get it back?" Tennis couldn't even be a consideration—what was I thinking? I had to be able to do just that one exercise. It seemed so simple that I began to wonder how could I have been unable to do it.

I felt strongly that the one hour of physical therapy allotted each day wasn't enough time for me to master this activity. I had to practice, but I wasn't allowed to do so without a therapist. Thus, began my practice of illegal exercise.

The privacy curtains that could be drawn around my bed were crucial to my illicit scheme. If Dawn had caught wind of this, I doubted whether she would have been surprised. But nonetheless, I had to make sure she didn't know.

I always awoke at the crack of dawn. With the exception, perhaps, of a brief nursing procedure, nothing much happened until the aides began delivering breakfast trays about an hour later.

I made sure that the privacy curtain was pulled all the way around me, which effectively concealed my bed from the view of anyone in the hallway. Next, I pressed the bedside control button that raised the head of my bed nearly to the vertical position. This provided support. Then, I turned myself over, pulling my nearly useless body around by gripping hold of the bed rails. That alone was arduous exercise.

Once I attained the kneeling position, I caught my breath and began. Just as in therapy, I lowered myself to the sitting position while holding onto the bed rails for balance and support. Then I forced myself to hold the position for as many seconds as I could—usually ten. After just two or three repetitions, I began to feel faint. Then, I swung myself around again and lay back to recover. I did this drill as many times as I could, but I always remembered to conserve enough energy for my morning shower. If Dawn ever knew, and I suspect that she did, she never let on.

There were some activities that I was allowed to do on my own. One was bridging, in which I lay on my back with my feet flat, then tried to raise my legs and pelvis. Leg lifts, from a sitting position, were another. Unless I absolutely needed to rest, I was always moving my feet and arms and trying to sit up. I exercised anything I could move, and I exercised until my eyelids drooped.

I am certain this helped me progress. My body learned to have success, and this, in turn, I believe, led to more success.

Around the end of June, just weeks after my admission to Spaulding as a quadriplegic, my therapists started to work, in earnest, on my walking. One morning, Dawn suddenly announced, "We're going to do something different today. I'm taking a chance. This may not work. You might not be ready for it just yet, but let's give it a try."

I certainly was game. I was willing to try anything that would bring me closer to walking again. This next order of business was something called the standing table. I was wheeled over to the new contraption in my chair, which was then locked firmly in place. A harness was buckled around my hips to hold me in place. Next, I reached forward, got a grip on the arms of the wheelchair, and tried to heave myself—claw my way up, actually—into a standing position. While in this standing position, I leaned forward against an inflatable form molded to the shape of my legs while I supported my arms on a wide, chest-level shelf.

The idea was to practice standing for as long as possible, which wasn't easy. Despite the supports, I became dizzy and lightheaded just raising myself into position. But, I managed to do it. The first time, I stood for two full minutes before needing to catch my breath and rest. I could tell I had made some sort of progress by the smiles of the therapists.

I didn't understand how and when this would add up to walking again. But two days later, the weekend therapists put me on the standing table for a second time. That day, I was able to raise myself into position without using the harness, and stood for a whopping three minutes without succumbing to fatigue or dizziness. Again, the therapists seemed to be amazed at the progress.

The next order of business was my stance. There was much to remember—to relearn—in order for me to achieve the proper stance in preparation for walking. I had to relax my shoulders and align them over the hips, which should be over the knees, which should be over the ankles, with feet not too close together, nor knees too close together, either.

This was tough, slow business. But I had to get that stance right. Otherwise, the walking wouldn't happen. First, I had to practice standing. Focusing so intently on all the nuances of a proper stance, which I never had

had to think of before, took all of my concentration. Then, and only then, would I actually be able to move.

The therapists' refrain was, "Lean slightly forward, tummy tucked in, everything in the proper alignment and relax. Now, walk."

Dawn's favorite reprimand was, "Don't rest on your ligaments!" This scold was repeated often by my champion therapist, who never seemed to let up.

The standard issue walker was next on my agenda. Laboriously, I lifted the device, moved it forward, set it down, carefully took a small step, then lifted it again as I began the sequence again, and again, and again after that. Slowly, tediously, and haltingly, I made my awkward way around Spaulding's gym. I tried hard to get the diagonal rotation from one leg to the other. This is a natural movement that one never thinks about, but it was surprisingly difficult to purposefully coordinate. All the while, I attempted to relax and achieve a semblance of normal movement. In order to make it work, I concentrated on everything and tried to remember it all.

"You're so stiff," the therapists complained.

But, I was walking. However awkwardly, I was walking.

I got down to the pier to exercise as often as I could. I always felt better being outdoors. I would park my wheelchair at one of the benches, lock the chair in place, and do leg lifts. One afternoon, Janice Higgins, my weekend therapist, spotted me from the fourth floor and came down.

"One of my patients has canceled," she said. "Would you like an extra session today?"

"You bet," I said eagerly.

We zoomed upstairs as fast as those wheels could go and, with Janice's superb coaching, I had an excellent, surprisingly exciting session. At the end of the bonus session, she placed her two strong hands, like bookends, on my chest and back to steady me, then guided me down the hall. The date was July 3, and I was walking down the corridor, strong and steady, with Janice's help and without a device.

◆ ◆ ◆

July 4, 1998, was noteworthy not only for the fireworks over the Esplanade in Boston, but for the single worst night of my stay at Spaulding Rehab. Exhausted, I fell sound asleep at 8:30 PM. Forty-five minutes later, my roommate, Miss May, a sweet, confused, ninety-six-year-old stroke victim, began talking, to no one in particular, in her native Chinese. Nurses tried to calm her to no avail. The loud, disruptive monologue went on until 2:30 in the morning, when the nurses finally wheeled her bed out of our room and into the solarium. I was so upset that I had chest pains. The nurses checked me out and monitored the situation closely. The pains, probably just gastrointestinal upset, ultimately dissipated, but not before prompting visions of my going back to Beth Israel-Deaconess with a heart problem.

When the nurses arrived for my 6:00 AM procedure, I was more exhausted than ever and distraught. My urgency to get better, coupled with the knowledge that I needed every ounce of strength I could muster, made me realize that just a single sleepless night could translate into a setback. The look on my face prompted immediate expressions of sympathy from the nurses, and that, in turn, drew tears of frustration on my part. Sympathy always did me in. It was one of the few times that I broke down in the hospital.

During my physical therapy session with Janice that morning, I related the events of the night before and the wee hours of that morning. "I'm just not sure," I explained, "what I'll be able to do today."

"We can work on some things that won't tax your energy too much," she said.

After setting me up on the walker, I hobbled in my usual fashion around the gym. Then I did a few exercises on the raised mat. At the end of our session, she brought my wheelchair around. I prepared to transfer into it so I could return to my room.

But Janice had other ideas.

"Stand up and hold onto the chair," she quietly commanded, as she set the wheelchair in front of me, facing outward. "Put your hands on the back of the handles, and stay close to it."

I was game, but had no idea what was about to happen. As instructed, I walked my wheelchair the length of the gym and out the door.

"Now turn right and keep going," Janice said.

"Okay," I said. Excitement was beginning to bubble.

The most magnificent feeling came over me: I was *walking*. Walking in this manner, pushing a vehicle on wheels was so fluid and natural. It was the best walking experience of my rehab career to this point.

"It's just like pushing a baby carriage," I exclaimed.

By the time I traversed the first two corridors outside the gym and entered the third, which led to my room, I might as well have been walking on air. It was the most real sensation, the closest thing to actual walking that I had done at Spaulding Rehab. I was elated and so were my pals on the fourth floor. They stopped. They beamed. They clapped their hands in pure delight. When Teresa McLaughlin saw me walking, her jaw dropped. She shook her head and began to cry. Janice cried, and I cried, too—tears of happiness, of course.

Shortly after I completed my little journey that morning, Bruce and the children arrived. So I made the trip all over again for the photographers, my family and new Spaulding pals. This time, I was the one giving my children a ride in my wheelchair. It was especially joyous for me to see the looks of delight and amazement on the faces of B.G. and the kids. It was a triumph I'll never forget.

◆ ◆ ◆

Physician's progress notes:

July 6, 1998

Attending: Patient in excellent spirits [and] pleased with continued rapid recovery. Pelvic control improved.

—J. Stein, MD

July 7, 1998

Attending: Mobility continues to improve … Needs cues to slow down, especially when turning … Caloric counts good.

—J. Stein, MD

The next big step in my recovery process was the removal of the PEG tube, which had been my main conduit for food during the time I was comatose and for several weeks thereafter. I had been able to ingest soft, pureed food, and then regular food, through the normal channel for some time. However, the doctors needed to be sure I was gaining enough sustenance by that route before they could give the okay to remove the tube.

The removal of the PEG tube was a significant step in the recovery process, and it certainly felt significant. When resident fellow Dr. Adam Agranoff literally pulled the plug out of my stomach, it hurt like hell. But only for a moment.

Dr Stein authorized and oversaw the procedure. "One of my roles in rehabilitation," he told me, "is as 'the remover of tubes.' Many patients arrive with tracheostomy tubes, Foley [urinary] catheters, IV tubes, and PEG tubes. Each time a tube is removed, it is a step toward recovery."

I believe I had had them all.

July 8, 1998

Attending: Patient eating well with excellent tolerance of Ensure-Plus supplements. PEG tube removed at bedside today without difficulty … Catheter volumes high. [Patient] admits to excessive drinking despite not feeling thirsty—advised to reduce intake.

—J. Stein, MD

When you began to recover slight strength and range of motion, we were relieved, but still pessimistic about whether you would ever function at the same level you had been at before the illness. We were extremely surprised as you began your recovery, and each new gain was met with a sense of reservation about future gains. Despite our pessimism … every day, there seemed to be a new progression.

—P. Sandhu, MD

♦ ♦ ♦

None of my friends from my years at the University of Michigan knew what had happened. During the Fourth of July weekend, I had called Sue Hitchcock, my best pal from college. After gallivanting around the world, Hitch had finally settled down with her husband and their young daughter in New York City, just down the Eastern Seaboard from me.

"Wendel," she said. "What a great surprise. What's up?"

Hitch and I had been sorority sisters at the Kappa Kappa Gamma house where we had such fun. We were goofy and rebellious. We had wonderful dinner conversations where we bandied about our youthful ideals and goals, and then we cut up. We had a ball; nothing bothered us. We were notorious jokers and shared great, good fortune, healthy ambition, and good humor. It seemed as though we had the best of everything in those years. We were even well matched in sports. Hitch was the only woman who could beat me at squash, but it was always close.

Because of those memories, relating my story to Hitch turned out to be difficult in a way I hadn't anticipated. Thus far, I had been able to discuss discrete aspects of the event with composure. But when speaking with her, the wonderful adventures and unbridled hopes of that earlier life flooded over me and collided with what had just happened and all of its uncertainty. I was undone. During our challenging, sometimes halting conversation, my story overwhelmed me. There were moments when I simply couldn't speak, and didn't—because I didn't want Hitch to know I was weeping.

Less than one week after that conversation and the removal of the PEG tube, Hitch strode into my hospital room. With a cheerful, triumphant smile on her face, she carried a big, juicy filet mignon from The Palm and a bagful of treats from her Manhattan spa. She looked exactly as I had remembered, and we had such fun catching up.

Months later, Hitch wrote of the feelings that were prompted by that phone call.

December 22, 1998

Dear Wendel,

The reason I responded to your call last summer by going up to Boston was due to what I felt to be the mixed emotions of what you were telling me. On one hand, in your bravery & charm, you were sharing the strength and positive attitude about what you had been through. During this, emotion was tumbling out through the tears, which suggested another story. I didn't know if you were reaching into the past, to a place where things were simple & safe. I came up to be that safe place in case you needed an extra push into a full recovery...

Upon arriving, I could see I wasn't needed in that way—you were doing just fine, and I was only too happy to make a festive occasion of the visit. It was fun to see you regally host the gathering...

Love,

Sue

Only the best of old pals could understand precisely what was happening in my heart and soul during that conversation back in July. Perhaps she understood even better than I did.

The day Hitch arrived was one of the most special of days at Spaulding. That night was an evening of old friends, new friends, family, and optimism. Hitch had arrived in the middle of a visit from Jessica Brown. Jessica and I had met in the back pew of the Unitarian Church in Newburyport where we sat with our newborn infant daughters. After Jessica left, Bruce showed up with the children, and I was delighted that Hitch could see B.G. again and meet Westy and Lindsay. Then Foster came. A little while later, another colleague from John Hancock appeared with Marisa Morin in tow.

◆ ◆ ◆

For as long as she could remember, Marisa had been what she came to understand as a psychic. Well regarded as a medical intuitive and healer, she had received plaudits for her work with medical research doctors and with high-risk teens. Although Marisa's expertise seemed a bit off the beaten path, I was open to anything that might help me reclaim my life.

Marisa was almost dismissive of her extraordinary abilities. "It was nothing I thought about or even wondered about," she wrote me later. "I assumed the whole world was having the same experiences."

Her letter continued:

I work with the soul of the person I am with, whether I'm in the same room or thousands of miles away. That is how I access information. When I am "scanning" someone, I can see his or her soul story written in that person's body and energy field, which are one and the same. Parts of this story are important to healing. I act as an interface among the soul, the psyche, and the body by communicating to the conscious mind what is present. The conscious mind can then integrate fully into the picture that is present, face the proverbial shadow, and integrate the energy that is there.

Technically speaking, I am clairaudient, clairsentient, and clairvoyant. I can see, hear, and feel a scene someone experienced at two years of age that is stuck in the body somewhere, usually in the form of a limiting belief. I can hear instructions from my own "guide" or someone else's. Occasionally, this comes as a voice, but most often, it is a knowing. I just know, or realize, what the guide is saying. This particular form of communication occurs a lot when I am doing medical readings.

Every once in awhile, someone calls me to contact someone who has died. This work is quite different. Most often, these folks come to me as they appeared in their lives. I think this is to prove to their loved ones that they are still alive, in a sense.

One of my favorite contacts from this realm was with a man who wanted to convey just one message to his loved ones: that he had a Ford truck. So he showed up with his shiny, new Ford truck. I could see every detail. I described it to his family, and they were deeply moved.

The man was a lifelong employee of General Motors and had, indeed, always secretly wanted to own a Ford.

After Foster and Bruce and the children left, Marisa offered to work on me. I would later refer to the evening of Marisa's visit as my tribal night.

"Sure," I agreed, not knowing what to expect. I thought that perhaps she would ask me some questions, synthesize the answers, and produce a report. Instead, something else happened.

"I am going to use an ancient Oriental technique to access your energy fields," she said as she approached me where I lay. "Stay just as you are: relax."

She started her work. With her strong, but gentle hands, she began at the back of my neck and gently bore down, her fingers pressed together much as if she were giving me a relaxing, as opposed to arduous, massage. Concentrating, she did not speak. She moved her hands down my back, arms, and legs. After a while, she began to shake her head slowly back and forth with obvious incredulity.

"This is amazing," she finally said. "This is fascinating. I have never experienced working with anyone with a neurological disorder before. Your body has tremendous energy. It's as though your body is learning from itself how to heal itself—and it's learning very quickly."

Then she said something startling, "You have the energy of a healer."

"What does that mean?" I asked

"If you had been born into a Native American tribe a hundred years ago, your gift would have been recognized by an elder of the tribe. You would have been taken to the shaman, the medicine man, to learn the healing ways of the tribe—midwifery and the like. You probably have had this effect on people your whole life and not realized it."

While Marisa gave me my gentle Oriental massage and wondered at *my* supposedly amazing healing power, I was given a pedicure: pink toenails for the first time in decades. Dear old Hitch, meanwhile, ever open to creativity and new ideas, simply sat off to one side, her eyes closed, a restful little smile on her pretty and familiar face. Then they all plucked rose petals from one of the flower arrangements lining the windowsill and sprinkled them over my body, like a blessing. The soft light of the setting sun gradually gave way to dusk and then nightfall. Our evening together, the women of the fold coming to the aid of the ailing one, came to an end.

Months later, Marisa wrote to me that she had been aware of my situation when I was first taken to Beth Israel-Deaconess, before the onset of my coma.

She wrote that the "intention of my visit was for me to serve your soul in any way that I was asked to." She explained:

When I arrived, I understood that I was to assist you in integrating your experience, which was profoundly spiritual, with your body conscious. I was aware that there had been quite a lot of bio-electrical challenges for you as a result of your adventures.

I met Foster, Bruce and the children, and your most amazing friend, Hitch. It was perfect. Their energy gave me quite a bit of information about what was happening with you and, perhaps more importantly, what energy of yours you shared with them. They were your tribe.

I remembered that at the beginning of that July evening, when everyone was still there, Marisa had sat by me for a long time, quietly observing, simply taking in her surroundings. She later wrote:

In essence, I was balancing the energy that was there—communicating that there would be healing in that space. I heard your soul clearly … You had a tremendous spiritual awakening and took a quantum leap of spiritual evolution. Some would call it an epiphany. In fact, you were blasted, bio-electrically, out of your old paradigms, beliefs, and structures. A tremendous rebirth has occurred in your body, mind, and spirit. There is a very real connection to life and oneness that you have never recognized before. You became fully aware, and now you want to share your soul and life. All the ways that you previously gave your power away, to structures, systems, and even to people, have been restructured by your illness. You had to learn to receive. Your connection to source was renewed.

That night served as an interface between your soul and body. I helped your body to re-assimilate, to adjust to this new, higher frequency of energy that it was carrying. I worked with your major energy centers: chakras. They are the body's computers. Together, we opened the doors to balanced communication with your cells.

Marisa added that the Ancients, the wise ones of any antiquarian culture, would call what I had a waking journey. She continued:

You died and went home to God, but brought that experience back within your body. You experienced seeing God and bringing God back into your body in the middle of life, not at the end of life, as most people finally experience God, when they die. That night in the hospital, you were absolutely filled with light and bursting with soul energy. Your body was so super receptive to me. Although you still had memory in your soul, the memory in your cells had to be forged anew. There is this sheer, pure energy coursing through you. It is very beautiful, very different. This power you now must honor.

Marisa explained that my neurological recovery, getting the messages to again move between my brain and my body, was somewhat inhibited at the time of my tribal night. But because of the energy present in my body and the connections she helped forge, my recovery process was now freed to move along at breakneck speed.

Marisa later wrote: *I also experience guides, or angels. They do not appear to me with wings, or degrees of mastery. Instead, they come and sit with me, much as I did with you in the hospital, and we have a conversation. It is indeed love that is the fabric of the universe. I know it is love that enables me to do this work. It is the eternal love of the soul that connects all of us to the truth of our oneness with all that is and all that ever will be.*

◆ ◆ ◆

Next on the agenda, I wanted Mel.

Despite fatigue, I was doing much better. And if it took my last ounce of energy, I would break out to see Mel.

Mel Ryan became well known at Spaulding. Long before I could travel any distance, let alone to the North Shore, I spoke longingly of visiting her, obviously thinking of the psychological lift I'd get from a visit to my favorite salon. My entreaties, impossible and illogical at first, finally worked. I made it to Mel's on July 11. Bruce came to Spaulding with the children to receive a lesson (again, required), from Janice, my favorite weekend therapist, on how to support me as I walked with a cane. Then we were off.

It was my first visit home since I had become ill, and it seemed otherworldly. I felt like a visitor in my own car, so familiar yet so foreign. It was wonderful to be sitting with the children, trying to keep Lindsay entertained in the back seat of the car, just like old times. After the heavy rains of June, the marshes of the North Shore looked more lush and green than ever. Being away from the hospital environment heightened all my senses. I felt a bit overwhelmed by the rich emerald greenery and moist air. The world almost seemed too beautiful.

I did not go into our house. I decided that it would have been too unsettling to have to leave it and return to the hospital. We just pulled into the driveway briefly to pick up a present for a birthday party that Westy was attending. We then drove to the party. Bruce walked Westy inside while Lindsay and I remained behind before going to Mel's.

Physician's progress notes:

July 13, 1998

Upper extremities strength much improved; lower extremities still weak, but better ... Neuropsychiatry testing today ... Home visit this week ... Predriving evaluation ordered.

—A. Agranoff, MD

Neuropsychiatry: Evaluation in progress.

Performance to date is encouraging re: return to work.

—W. Klein. PhD

Four days later, I talked to Westy on the phone, from the hospital. The next day, July 16, was his eighth birthday, and it didn't look as though I would be able to make it to his party at the Oldtown Club. Kate was with me, waiting to start my afternoon exercise session. I explained to Westy that I couldn't get away from the hospital for any length of time. I didn't want both Bruce and me to miss Westy's party, for Bruce would have had to chauffeur me the considerable round-trip distance.

Full of false cheer, I said, "Westy, when I get home, we'll have another party, even better than the first."

"Okay ..." he said, his little voice drifting off, stoic and accepting. Though he didn't complain, I could hear his disappointment.

At my end, I had begun to weep. "I love you, honey," I said. "I'll miss you."

"I'll miss you, too, Mom."

Well, that did it. I was undone, in tears. I hung up the phone and turned to Kate. "I'm sorry," I said. "I'll be all right in a minute. I just have to do something about this."

After we finished my exercises, I zoomed down the hall in my wheelchair to see the doctors, nurses, and therapists to figure out how to solve my problem.

By coincidence, the therapists had scheduled a visit to our house the following morning to assess how I might move around in it after my discharge. Could I go with them and stay the day? No, that wouldn't work because of other therapy schedules at the hospital. I pitched the nurses and doctors with another idea, and they agreed. Because I was doing so well with my procedures, they said they would set me up for the day.

I went to the house with the therapists in the morning, stayed for Westy's party—I couldn't imagine how it would have felt to miss it—and made plans to leave the children with a favorite sitter before returning to the hospital with Bruce the same evening.

Before leaving the house for the club, I tossed a swimsuit in my bag, just in case. I remembered that weeks before, when I had only just begun to show signs of improvement, Dr. Stein said I was a prime candidate for hydrotherapy. He was right. It was a glorious day, and it felt fabulous to be in the water in the pool of our little club. Everyone swam, and the kids were so happy. Westy remembered to call his buddies by name and thank each one as he opened his presents. It was a perfect summer birthday afternoon.

I felt so lucky—and grateful—to be there.

◆ ◆ ◆

From the time of my initial triumphs with the walkers, my progress was surprisingly swift and dramatic. By mid-July, I had progressed to a cane, but the therapists refused to leave one with me after my sessions. They rightly thought that I would try to do too much.

"It's nothing eight bucks wouldn't solve," Foster quipped one evening.

"If I had a cane brought in," I explained, "they would just take it away."

My next order of business was climbing stairs, which I was especially eager to do. We lived on three floors in a quirky charmer of a house with a floor plan that had been evolving, willy-nilly since the 1740s.

First, I climbed half a flight of stairs at the hospital, and the following day a whole flight of stairs and back down. Then I did two flights up and down, then four flights down to Spaulding's basement and the treadmill. I did all this slowly and cautiously. Then I ventured onto the treadmill.

One warm summer day, my therapists took me outside. "Today," Dawn announced, "I'm going to have you practice walking on uneven terrain." Just as we stepped outside, a friend, Greg Szumowski, showed up with a big bouquet of freshly cut flowers from his wife Linda's garden. He stayed for the entire therapy session, even though I couldn't carry on much of a conversation.

"Sorry, Greg," I apologized. "I can't walk and talk at the same time!" I had to concentrate on every single aspect of my stance and movement.

On another morning, later that week, Dawn found me standing unaided at the sink, brushing my teeth. "Aha! I caught you!" she scolded. As I started to defend myself, she made a glorious announcement. "I actually came to tell you that you have just gotten your independent walking status," she said, beaming with pride.

Happy day! This meant that I could legally walk anywhere in the hospital without a cane, or walker, or wheelchair. On this particular day, two friends, Cathy Ebling and Janet O'Hara, had come down from the North Shore for lunch. They went to my room and found it empty. What a thrill it was to greet them as I walked back from speech therapy without any assistance.

I'll never forget the looks of amazement and delight as they saw me, walking toward them that day.

Physician's progress notes:

July 17, 1998

> Urologic issues still need to be assessed ... Bath/Dressing—Distant supervision ... Meal prep—Distant supervision ... Some impulsiveness with quick movements ... Good lower extremities strength ... Somewhat impulsive behavior ... Needs home services ... Good gains [in] speech/cognitive improvement ... Physical therapy two times per week at home; no occupational therapy ... Has nanny, nursing two times per day.
>
> —A. Agranoff, MD

At each successive patient care conference (PCC), my estimated discharge date was moved up further and further. When I arrived at Spaulding on June 9, recently comatose and quadriplegic, my length of stay was estimated at twelve weeks. No signs of progress were anticipated until December, if then. Now my discharge was scheduled for July 20.

It was odd in a way. As my discharge date drew near, I had a heightened awareness of having lived another life at Spaulding. Now I was about to "cross over" from the wheelchair-bound world to the walking world, where perhaps I would not feel so special any longer. I was leaving a place, and a way of life, that had unexpectedly become very familiar for a time, but one to which, God willing, I would not return.

◆ ◆ ◆

It is said of Boston's Spaulding Rehabilitation Hospital that people are carried in the front door, and they walk out the back door. I was carried in the side door, but walked out the front, hewing, in the end, to the Spaulding legend.

Physician's progress notes:

July 17, 1998

> Patient self-cathing without difficulty ... Ambulating independently ... Home visit yesterday went well ... Neurology: upper extremities strength much improved; lower extremities still weak, but better ... Neuropsychiatry testing-formal report pending. No obvious cognitive deficits ... Anticipate discharge on July 20.
>
> —A. Agranoff, MD

My discharge evaluations were uniformly joyous, triumphant, and poignant. My speech therapist, Denise Ambrosio, ended hers by asking me to write a few paragraphs about my experience at Spaulding. She wanted to check my vocabulary and grammar, but she also wished to see if I could organize my thoughts. In one way, the essay was an easy exercise. My experience was so profound and miraculous that no embellishment was needed. But, and this I had not anticipated, it was also an emotional challenge. I wrote just a little more than a page, and it took only twenty minutes. But I used up several tissues in the process.

Denise read it and was openly moved. She asked my permission to share the essay with the staff, which I was glad to do. I wanted people to know how important they were.

> *When I was admitted to Spaulding on June 9, I was quadriplegic, although I didn't realize how impaired I actually was. This inaccurate realization was, I believe, beneficial, for I would not have wanted to be discouraged as I set out to make myself whole again ...*
>
> *I began my road to recovery by flopping in a wheelchair. I was told that, in order to walk [again], I would first have to learn to sit and*

then stand with balance. I didn't know how I was going to do this, but I was determined, early on, to go home without a wheelchair.

Therapy was incredibly arduous in the early days and weeks. I was not strong, and I was quite impaired. But I had to get better. I have two beautiful young children, a wonderful husband, and an incredible network of family, friends, and colleagues. I also have a great job at an excellent company. I wanted my life back, but most of all, I missed my children. They were my great motivation.

Physical, occupational, and speech therapists worked with me daily to restore the abilities that were damaged by ADEM and twelve days in a coma. Miraculously, progress was swift and sometimes dramatic. Activities and exercises that were difficult on a Monday were easier by Tuesday or Wednesday. I can't say enough in praising the Spaulding staff for their talent, caring, and encouragement. Thanks to these people, I will walk out of here on Monday, July 20, with my family.

On that last Sunday at Spaulding, July 19, Janice conducted my discharge evaluation for physical therapy. She checked my strength and abilities against my baseline measurements at the time of my admission and made the appropriate comparative notes. Then she brought me into the hallway.

"There are two more things I want you to do," she said, with a hint of mischief. "I want you to skip down the hall."

"Skip?" I asked, incredulous.

"Skip," she confirmed. "Go ahead. See what you can do."

Well, I did it, although it felt like I was carrying a sack of potatoes.

"Okay, that was good," Janice said. "Now, there's one more thing I want you to do. Run down the hall."

"Run?" I asked, incredulous as before.

"Run."

Hesitating only momentarily, wondering if I could actually do what Janice had asked, I picked up one foot, gave it a little lift, and with that first little jump, propelled myself forward into, yes, a run. A plodding, but exciting run. I was very much out of shape, and I had a keen sense of the force of gravity. My limbs felt extremely heavy. But I was, indeed, running down the hall where I'd been pushed, flopping in a wheelchair, to my first physical therapy session not six weeks earlier.

Five weeks and five days after my admission to Spaulding, quadriplegic after nearly dying, I skipped and ran unaided down the fourth-floor corridor of my soon-to-be vacated residence. When I told B.G. about it, he chuckled in delight—and amazement.

It seemed as though a miracle had occurred, indeed.

♦ ♦ ♦

July 20, 1998, dawned bright and sunny. It would be a happy, hectic, and exciting morning. For the last time, Constantine brought me my favorite Spaulding breakfast: oatmeal, cranberry juice, and a double order of blackened bacon. As he handed me my tray, I said goodbye. "Thank you, Constantine. You have done so much for me. I'll never forget you."

He reached for my hand to give me a strong but gentle handshake. "You take care, Ford," his typical, abbreviated greeting, delivered with warmth and pride.

Then the phone rang. It was Foster, making his last early morning call to me in the hospital. It seemed an oddly dramatic moment. I suppose it might have been the symbolic finality of that last hospital call that caught me off guard—or perhaps the beginning of a new chapter. But it caught me by surprise.

After breakfast, my caregivers started coming around. Lee, Kate, and Brenda from Occupational Therapy stopped by. Dawn pushed herself to come in for the goodbye, even though she was feeling under the weather. Janice was there. Dr. Stein and Dr. Agranoff came by to wish me well as did the aides and nurses who were beaming proudly. There was so much warmth, love, and gratitude. Someone from the development office stopped by to ask if the hospital could use my story. I was so busy saying goodbye that Francine, one of my favorite aides, took it upon herself to empty my little closet and pack my bags.

B.G. and the children arrived, and Westy snapped lots of happy pictures of the staff with their miracle patient

We were all so happy, and then we were off.

♦ ♦ ♦

I shall never forget my first morning home. I awoke and slowly made my way up the stairs to Lindsay's nursery on the third floor. She was standing in her crib. Smiling, her eyes sparkling, she had a look of delighted wonderment on her face. Momentarily drinking in the scene, I said nothing.

We just fell in love with each other all over again, and it was rapturous. I took her in my arms, both of us giggling softly, and picked up, so I hoped, where we had left off.

I was warned that coming home might be more traumatic than I had anticipated, and in some ways it was. It was reaffirming to have walked out of the hospital and then to be with my family. But I was exhausted. I looked normal, but I was as depleted as a functioning person could be. I realized early on how much I needed sustenance upon waking in the morning. I found that if I drank a can of Ensure and a bit of Gatorade, I could get around to such simple renewed joys as making beds and tending to the children. On most days, I was fatigued around 9:30 in the morning. But by late morning, I typically got a second wind, which enabled me to drive to our little country club for a day of swimming and rest.

I swam laps daily for the rest of the summer, in one- to two-hour sessions between twenty and fifty minutes each. In between, I rested by the pool, watched the children, and visited with friends. I lunched on the porch and otherwise had a true country club summer, something I had never allowed myself before—at least not to that extent. By summer's end, Lindsay could swim on her own, and I, too, was much improved. Without having to buck gravity, I was able to exercise my atrophied muscles and regain much of my lost strength. The pool was a Godsend.

After Labor Day, the pool closed and Lindsay began nursery school. For the first time in nine years, I was kid-less and not pregnant. I immediately called around to schedule tennis.

I had thought that with luck I would have the strength to be able to play tennis the following summer. But the doctors and therapists said I could try then. On September 10, 1998, I was back on the court with an understanding partner, Cynthia Brown.

It felt extraordinary. This was another milestone and, for a host of reasons, a major one. The day was beautiful and clear on the headland, which overlooked the Parker River, out toward Ipswich Bay and the Atlantic Ocean. The old clay courts held their reputation as the place where every bounce was an adventure. Though I was able to play again, I wasn't very good. I told B.G. that this was his big chance to wallop me at tennis, but he didn't take advantage. We were both just so happy and amazed to be back on the courts together, as though nothing had ever happened. Life was fine indeed.

Indeed, the milestones were never ending.

"You live near the beach, don't you?" asked Dr. Stein. "Walk the beach in your bare feet. It will be excellent exercise for you."

What a magnificent experience my winter beach was with all its restorative power. I had been down to Plum Island countless times with my family, but being there off-season, alone, was almost spiritual. Some days, I was on that glorious six-mile stretch of sand with not another soul in sight. Just me, the mist, and the sand dollars.

♦ ♦ ♦

My recovery had never been a foregone conclusion. Virtually all the medical people who came in contact with me—doctors, therapists, and nurses—were surprised that I was able to leave Spaulding within six weeks of my arrival, fully ambulatory. Some were shocked that I left at all.

Several weeks later, I received a letter from Dr. Stein. In it, he wrote:

> *Given the degree of disability you were experiencing when you arrived, we expected a protracted recovery and likely some persistent limitations. Happily, we were wrong ... I try to learn from every person I care for. The remarkable ability of the human body, and brain, to recover is something that I need to be reminded of when confronted with severe illness, and I frequently remind myself of your case when I have a new patient with severe problems.*

Dr. Thomas Scammell, the brilliant young research doctor from Harvard who headed my neurology team at Beth Israel-Deaconess, told me simply, "We don't often have outcomes like this from such dire beginnings."

"Your case was both surprising and inspiring," wrote Dr. Paul Sandhu, one of my attending physicians at Spaulding:

> *The natural tendency of physicians is to guard against becoming emotionally involved with their patients. This is particularly true when faced with a patient with dramatic and seemingly irreversible severe impairment. I have to say that, to date, I have never seen such a remarkable turn around in terms of neurological deficit ... Any recovery from complete ventilator-dependent quadriplegia to complete recovery is both extraordinary and miraculous ...*
>
> *Every physician loves to have a "miracle case" like this one.*

But perhaps the most dramatic response came from Dr. David Trentham, the rheumatologist at Beth Israel-Deaconess. Nine months after my discharge, I e-mailed him, along with several others:

> *Dear Dr. Trentham, perhaps you remember my case. I was hospitalized in Beth Israel-Deaconess's medical intensive care unit last May and June with ADEM. Fortunately, I made what has been referred to as a miraculous recovery, thanks to all of you at the BIDMC and Spaulding*

Rehab in Boston. I have begun to write about my medical adventure, and I must ask you for your help ...

Dr. Trentham's hastily e-mailed reply: *"Poor typist, will call. Can,t believe your alive. David Trentham."*

It was clear to me that surviving a coma was an extraordinary experience. Having survived, I don't believe I ever felt quite so full of life. I have a deeper appreciation of everything in my life—especially the people in my life. Acquaintances became friends; friends became the best of friends; re-connections occurred with long-lost friends.

Sometimes, I was almost delirious at having recovered my life. I had come full circle from the first warning sign, the delirium in spring 1998, that I might have something more than the flu. Homely joys such as making the beds, working in the kitchen, and picking up after the children would never again be taken for granted. Kneeling on Westy's bed to raise the shade each morning never failed to remind me of the high-kneeling activity at Spaulding. It had been my Everest, my impossible goal. As I swam on my back at the health club, I looked up at the ceiling of the pool-house and recalled the feeling I had looking up at the ceiling in my hospital room, when I wondered if I might ever be the same again.

The memories were poignant. Just looking out the kitchen window at the garden or preparing breakfast for my children like any other suburban mom, memories of my other life, my hospital life, often flooded over me. I would think, as did Dr. Scammell at the height of the crisis, "There, but for the grace of God ..."

♦ ♦ ♦

In November 1998, I took Westy into Boston for a special weekend. The Massachusetts Institute of Technology (MIT) had accepted him for a two-day enrichment program, and we decided to do it up right. We took the train down and stayed with friends in our old Back Bay neighborhood. It felt good to be back—much like a homecoming.

I sprung for tickets to "The Blue Man Group," the creatively avant-garde musical hit, which Westy loved. We ate breakfast at the Copley Plaza—Westy was just old enough to appreciate the experience of the only palace hotel in Boston. We explored the Esplanade, studied the statuary on the Commonwealth Avenue mall, and I introduced him to the Boston Public Library.

Everyone we met, from our hosts to strangers at subway and bus stops, from the wait staff at the restaurants and stores to the folks at MIT and the theatre were, to a person, delightful. People seemed charmed at the sight of a mother and her young son on a city outing. Little could they know how special it truly was. Even the weather cooperated.

As Westy and I walked along the Esplanade, it struck me how our lives had changed from just a few months earlier. "Do you remember the last time we were here together, on the river?" I asked him.

"Yes …" said Westy, after a pause. "It was when you were at the hospital."

"That's right, honey," I replied. "Isn't it wonderful that I can *walk* here with you now, instead of sitting in a wheelchair on the Spaulding pier?"

Third in a line, like his Grandma Billie and his WowMom, Westy never doubted that I would recover.

As we walked along the river in the most wonderful city in the world, my little prince smiled up at me and said, "I thought you had at least a ninety-nine point one million ninths of a percent chance."

Part Three

"Your very desire to live and not die was itself a kind of prayer."

Professor Kimberley Patton, April 1999
Harvard Divinity School
Cambridge, Massachusetts

Chapter Eight

In Search of Meaning

Years after my near-death experience, the two central medical mysteries remained unsolved. Why did I get ADEM? And why did I recover from it so quickly and, apparently, so thoroughly?

The first question asked by nearly everyone who heard my story was, "Is it true they still don't know what caused this?"

The answer is yes. From the very beginning and over the course of several months, scores of tests were run, some repeatedly, pages and pages worth, at Beth Israel-Deaconess and at Spaulding. The blood that was taken from me nearly every day was sent to the National Centers for Disease Control in Atlanta, which did not accept cases unless their own research doctors were assured that all local resources had been exhausted in the quest for answers. Years later, there were no concrete answers.

While not a medical scientist, I was a researcher by profession, and I also knew myself fairly well. My hypothesis to explain the origins of my disorder is based on a combination of factors that more or less caused the planets to align against me:

- For a long while, I had been unusually fatigued. For someone who ate well, exercised regularly, did not suffer from depression, and hardly ever was sick, I went through a period of being terribly tired almost all the time for several years.
- I had been working in our garden, which included stacking the woodpile, with its old, partially fungal wood, just days before I fell ill.
- The week I succumbed, I'd had a bad sinus infection.
- Superimposed on all of this was an atypically high level of stress brought on by an unusual circumstance. On May 15, 1998, before lunch at Maison Robert with Bruce, we had attended an Immigration and Naturalization Service (INS) hearing. The INS had asked us to testify as

witnesses for them in the case of an illegal alien con artist who had used my children in an attempt to rob my family 18 months earlier.
- Coupled with an already weakened system, I strongly believed there was a good chance that the upsetting experience with the INS may have been the capping blow.

In August 1998, I began a course of outpatient physical therapy at our local hospital, where my medical adventure officially began three months earlier. I engaged in conversation with my new therapist, asking if she had ever before worked with anyone with a disorder similar to mine.

Her answer, of course, was no.

"Have you worked with anyone who has been in a coma?" I asked next.

This time, the answer was yes, twice. In both cases, the cause of the coma was stress.

◆ ◆ ◆

On December 13, 1996, a woman whom Bruce and I hoped would be our children's new nanny came to sit for Westy and Lindsay for three hours. Bruce and I planned to attend a benefit holiday art show just down the street from our home.

As was my habit, I covered a lot of ground over the telephone while interviewing this prospective nanny. With this method, I could usually weed out 98 percent of prospects. I carefully checked references. Only then did I ask Elizabeth N. to the house to meet Bruce, the children, and me. We spoke with her for several hours. We covered every aspect of care relating to the children. We discussed everything from love and discipline to diet, bath, and television. She explained her general philosophy of child care itself. She told me everything I wanted to hear.

And none of it would turn out to be true.

On December 13, 1996, she babysat for Westy and Lindsay. We gave her instructions to feed the children and get them to bed between 8:00 and 8:30 PM, which was their usual routine. We asked her to honor our policy of no television in the evening. She told us she wholeheartedly supported our no-TV approach.

When we returned at 10:00 that evening, all the lights were on and the two children were running around. Our six-year-old son had been left alone to watch a frightening rescue program. Twenty-two-month-old Lindsay had been left alone long enough for her to climb three floors by herself.

When I realized the extent to which this woman had neglected our children, disregarded the in-depth conversations we had had about how

Bruce and I wanted our children cared for, and generally deceived us, we dismissed her. It was nothing that we even had to discuss. B.G. and I were always on the same page with regard to the children, and we saw everything instantly. It was a terrible experience, but no real harm had come to them, although it could have. As the door closed behind her, B.G. and I breathed a sigh of relief that it was over.

But it was not over. While our children were being neglected, the sitter had been very attentive to our financial records. Ten days later, I learned that she had applied for a loan using me as a cosigner, complete with my work address and Social Security number.

After reporting this to the district attorney, Bruce and I began the long process of trying to undo the damage of the attempted identity theft. Ultimately, Ms. N. was tried, punished, and received a two-year suspended sentence. However, she violated her parole conditions and was sentenced to eighteen months.

Concurrent with the criminal proceedings, she was investigated by the Bureau of Immigration and Naturalization Service. Determined to keep this con artist away from other unsuspecting parents, Bruce and I agreed to testify on behalf of the INS at a bond hearing to determine whether Ms. N., a Ugandan, should be released from prison, and, if so, for how much bail.

The hearing was set for May 15, 1998.

Bruce and I arrived at the John F. Kennedy Federal Building at Government Center in Boston at the appointed hour. We were thoroughly briefed on the system and the procedures of the morning's hearing by a young INS lawyer. He then informed us that Ms. N. had been making potentially scandalous claims about some sort of "history" she'd had with Bruce. According to this lawyer, Ms. N. also asserted that it was Bruce who had encouraged her to steal my W-2 form that night in December 1996.

Bruce handled the session calmly, as usual. I, on the other hand, had never been more emotionally churned up at any time in my adult life. I could not think of a more unpleasant episode than the one that had unfolded as the result of our interaction with that woman. I was sickened that such a person could even be in our ken.

She stared at me menacingly throughout the entire hearing as I stated time after time for her court-appointed lawyer that it would have been impossible for my husband to know this woman at any time *ever*.

"How do you know?" he kept asking me.

"I just know," I answered, incredulous.

This exchange was repeated numerous times, until the INS lawyer finally protested. "Your honor, he's just badgering the witness."

The judge finally set cash bail at $20,000.

To put the unpleasantness of the morning behind us, B.G. and I made our way to Maison Robert for lunch, just up the street from Government Center in downtown Boston. It was a glorious spring day, warm enough for us to sit outside at the cafe and enjoy the elegant cuisine.

The rest of the day continued pleasantly enough. We drove back home to interview the second-grade teachers at Westy's school in preparation for his upcoming school year. We then returned home to our children. We had supper in the garden and enjoyed the view of the sailboats in the outer harbor. Then I read stories and sang lullabies to my children and put them to bed.

"Good night, honey-bun," I told Lindsay, as I tucked her into bed. To Westy, it was, "'Night, buddy. I love you."

It would be weeks before I saw either of them again.

I recount the INS episode because I wonder if the tumult in my heart that day was enough to put my body over the edge into a realm only God knew. Perhaps we will never understand the havoc an unspeakable upset can wreak. Dr. Scammell, for one, tended to discount the stress connection. He and the other doctors focus on the other mystery: my quick and apparently complete recovery from a death-door coma and quadriplegia.

◆ ◆ ◆

My father, Wendell Phillips Chapin, had died of a massive stroke at the age of seventy-eight in the spring of 1990—three months before my first child, Westy, was born. Dad had lived a great long life. He stayed in excellent shape and played tennis several times a week. But what heartbreaking timing. Being unable to share my children with their extraordinary grandfather had been the great sadness of my life. Dad was a gentleman of the first rank. A somewhat shy and truly good person, he was a beloved tennis coach and an excellent player in his own right and in his own day. He had taught me how to play the game and also how to behave on the tennis court and off. The only tennis trophy I ever kept was a silver plate for sportsmanship that was given to me at a tournament in Midland, Michigan, when I was sixteen years old.

Dad reared me as he did his two sons. I never felt any distinction between his approach to bringing up my brothers and his approach to guiding me through life. He even might have been more thorough and exacting with me. I never forgot a comment on appearances that he made when I was about fifteen and had no idea how I came across to people.

"You know," he said, "there are a lot of good-looking women in the world. But they often become soft because they don't develop other aspects of their persona."

This was his warning of the pitfalls of coasting through life on one's looks. Although I felt I was all knees and teeth and braces, I tucked away the advice for life. And I tried to remember to toss the ball high enough and get that good, fluid movement in my serve, to be ever striving for the "sweet spot" and to follow through at tennis—and to make it into the University of Michigan. But, most important of all, he taught me to be ready. He was a great father because he made me feel as if I could do anything I set my mind to.

That attitude certainly prepared me for my rehabilitation struggle, which no one could have predicted.

George Dow, another great friend from John Hancock and a racquet player who understood tennis and knew of my background, came to visit me toward the end of my stay at Spaulding. He suggested that I had a successful recovery because I had been in such good physical shape. I immediately told him, "George, it was the mindset that tennis gave me that made the difference—the competitive mindset."

And that was a gift from Dad.

During my last week at Spaulding, I awoke one morning with heavy tears. Early mornings in the hospital were always difficult, and this one was both difficult and unusual because I distinctly sensed the presence of my father. His presence was so strong that I actually turned to look up around the head of my bed. I saw no vision, nor heard any spoken words. His presence was subtle but distinct, but the message that came through was clear and strong. I understood immediately that I was out of the woods, that Dad loved me and was proud of me—and that he was *there*, right *there*, *with* me. The sense of his spirit was indescribably strong. I recognized his presence and understood his reassuring message.

And, yes, I have always believed in angels.

♦ ♦ ♦

So perhaps my late father helped in an inexplicable and mystical way. Certainly an extensive network of friends, social and professional, helped my recovery. People came out of the woodwork on this one. We—Bruce, the children, and I—received scores of the most heartfelt sentiments and offers of help, including many from people we hardly knew. Serendipitously, the entire episode drew us closer to many people we had enjoyed before only as acquaintances.

Onalee Cooke had moved to our neighborhood just a couple of years earlier with her husband, Tom, the well-known artist of *Sesame Street*. We had met only a handful of times socially. Yet they sent flowers, called, and wrote several notes and letters:

July 8, 1998

Dear Wendy,

6. Just a note to let you know we are thinking of you and praying for your complete recovery real soon. I want to telephone you but don't want to interrupt your day, which (I understand) is filled with therapy sessions. I'll try in the evening soon, though, and hope Bruce will feel free to telephone me if there is anything I can do for your or your children.

Come home soon!

Fondly,

Onalee and Tom Cooke

We knew Jim and Vicki Dyer only in passing through the church, our clubs, and mutual friends. Yet Vicki's sincere offer to help, especially with our children, was touching:

Dear Bruce,

I have heard ... that Wendy has been ill, but now recovering. I'm praying for her quick recovery, and also would be very glad to help you and the kids. I'm at home most of the time; can run errands, or babysit—here or your home. Or perhaps you just need a break.

I'll call in a few days to see if there is anything we can do.

Vicki Dyer

A woman I knew only from my commute into Boston wrote:

Dear Wendy,

I just wanted to let you know my thoughts are with you in this most difficult time for you and your family. I am sorry to hear the news, which Onalee Cooke told me. But I am comforted by the fact, in my brief conversations with you, what a strong spirit and person you are.

I wish you a speedy recovery. If there is anything I can do for you, Bruce, or your children, please know that I am here for you.

I will hold you in my heart. Take care.

With warmest regards,

Julie (from the bus!!)

The beat went on.

During a visit to Spaulding, Foster once asked if I ever cried. "I have my moments," I told him. The early morning hours at Spaulding were rough, a melancholy time of reflection during which, as I waited for breakfast, I wondered if I would ever be able to walk again, to be a fun, active mom again, to have the life I had led before. It was too early in the day to call anyone. No one was around to bear up for. There was nothing much going on during those bleak dawn hours except the vicissitudes of my aching heart.

Once Foster learned of this early morning sadness, I began to receive phone calls almost daily, as soon as the hospital switchboard opened for business. Those priceless talks helped so much to fill that almost unbearable void, brightening those sad hospital mornings and getting my day off to a better start.

And my visitors! It seemed as if there was a party in my room nearly every day at Spaulding. I never knew in advance who would come; it was always a wonderful surprise. I am convinced these visits truly helped buoy my recovery process.

Moreover, Spaulding was not an easy place to visit. It was hard to see so many people in such dire straits. I, too, often averted my gaze from neighboring rooms, even though for six weeks, that place was my second home. I gave my visitors a lot of credit simply for walking through the door.

I returned to work on November 16, 1998, six months to the day that I fell ill. I was welcomed back with beautiful flowers, beaming faces, open arms, and yet another party. I circulated an e-mail thank-you from the bottom of my heart to the great-hearted people on the fifty-fourth floor of the Hancock Tower and elsewhere in the company:

Dear Friends:

We often think that doctors will have all the answers, but we really stumped them … this summer. There was a time when they didn't know if I would make it, and I did. There was a time when they didn't know if I would be able to walk again, or talk, or even think again, let alone so quickly. But we surprised them on that one, too.

The doctors now use the word "miracle" when they talk about my case.

What they didn't know, but came to realize, was that I had some secret magic, and it was all of you.

The visits—you visited me by the cab-load. There was a party in my room every day! The phone calls, from earliest morning (probably my toughest time) through evening, were my lifeline. The flowers—for more than two months—fresh flowers filled my room. I received, literally, pounds of cards and letters—dear messages and wishes. The prayers, which I continue to hear about, were powerful and they worked.

I was so fortunate to have had the best of everything. I could never say enough about Beth Israel-Deaconess or Spaulding Rehab. The doctors, bless them, never gave up on me. They were dedicated, courageous, and brilliant.

But there was something more than medicine at work here. All of you buoyed my spirits with your care and warmth. It truly helped me get better, and I shall never forget. So, thank you.

It's wonderful to be back.

Wendy

◆ ◆ ◆

Chapter Nine

Prayer

After wrestling with a commitment to organized religion, B.G. and I finally decided to ally ourselves with the Unitarian church. We liked the new minister, Harold Babcock—I could actually follow his uplifting and provocative sermons. And we cherished the idea that our children would learn about the universe of religions, rather than having one school of thought presented as ultimate truth. We valued the general approach of the church, which emphasized simplicity, universality, and a benevolent humanism. It seemed like a true fit.

What cinched the decision for Bruce, we joked, was that the church closes down in July and August. Bruce preferred to find his God on an open sailboat. We came to cherish this church, as B.G. put it so well, "because it celebrates life every day"—which is certainly what he did. So this was our religious life.

After I returned to work, Tim Hollingworth, my colleague at John Hancock, once asked me if I were a pray-er—that is, one who prayed. I had to stop and think.

"I don't think I've ever prayed for myself," I answered.

However, I added that I did thank God repeatedly for visiting this affliction upon me and not upon my children.

I had gone to sleep for years with my hands clasped together, thanking God for my great good fortune—for B.G. and my children and their health and happiness. I prayed each night for help in keeping Westy and Lindsay safe and for the wisdom, strength, and patience to be WowMom.

I never took life for granted before my medical adventure. I always had the sense that if something were too wonderful, it might be lost. An aunt of mine used to say that I had the Scottish sense of doom, a prescient sentiment, in view of what happened.

Countless people wrote to Bruce and me, or told us in person, of their prayers. One month after my discharge from Spaulding, Bruce visited with his mother, Mary, who showed him a collection of prayers I had given her several years earlier. She pointed to a page that literally was worn out.

"This is the prayer I turned to again and again for Wendy," she said:

Our Lady of Mount Carmel

O, Most beautiful flower of Mount Carmel, fruitful one.
Splendor of Heaven
Blessed Mother of the Son of God
Immaculate Virgin
Assist me in this my necessity.

O, Star of the sea
Help me and show me herein
You are my mother.

O, Holy Mary, Mother of God,
Queen of Heaven and earth,
I humbly beseech you
From the bottom of my heart
To succor me in this necessity;
There are none that can withstand your power.

O, show me herein you are my Mother.
O, Mary, conceived without sin,
Pray for us.
Who have recourse to thee.

Sweet Mother, I place this cause in your hands.

I had a poignant conversation with Anne Constable, my sister-in-law. Her father, John Constable, passed away while I was writing these memoirs. She told me her father had prayed for me.

My nephew Nick Springer and his classmates in Croton-on-Hudson, New York, prayed for me. My brother Robbie's church in Michigan prayed for me. A colleague of Bruce's who traveled in Europe that summer lit candles for me in every church she visited. The church of my sister-in-law, Nancy Springer, had a prayer circle for me. Foster's assistant, the beloved Paula Santosuosso, prayed to Saint Anthony and lit countless candles.

While I was in the coma, Bruce's sister-in-law, Terri Ford, another devout Catholic, obtained water from Lourdes and sprinkled it over me in the intensive care unit at Beth Israel-Deaconess, but not before visiting her parish priest to learn the ritual.

How did all of this happen and to what effect?

Professor Kimberly Patton, a friend who is a religious historian at Harvard Divinity School, was emphatic about her belief in the power of prayer. In the midst of writing this book, I asked her to comment:

April 10, 1999

Dear Wendy,

Thank you for sharing the section of the memoir you are writing about your extraordinary experience not even one year ago ... I think the urgency you feel to record what happened to you last year is part of a calling. Your story has already transformed you and will continue to do so. But it is also something that could transform others. I admire you tremendously for undertaking the task of writing. (The Quran, the holy book of Islam, was virtually dictated by the angel Gabriel to the Prophet Muhammed; the angel commanded him, "Write!" In a way, your angel is doing the same, and you are doing just the right thing by listening.)

You asked me if I could contribute something about prayer. I am hesitant to do so because I know so little about it and am such an erratic practitioner of prayer, even though Saint Paul enjoins us to "pray without ceasing." I am not a theologian but a historian of religion. But I am a fellow human being, and I have surely known despair in my life. And I have prayed, in fear or desperation, with all my heart, "foxhole prayers" ... Now I am learning to pray with trust and hope. "Thy will be done."

The only thing I do know and feel, as I said to you last summer, is that prayer works, and not just in the sense of helping the one who prays. It also helps the one who is prayed for. And it strengthens God's loving kindness, like pumping blood through a heart. The Muslims have a word for it; barakah, *meaning "blessing," "grace," or "holiness." Prayer circulates* barakah *through the arteries of the universe ...*

In reading the section you gave me to look at, I am struck by its beauty, honesty, and simplicity. I feel that in the tremendous suffering you endured, and in some ways, the even worse suffering that your family and friends endured as they waited to see if God would let you live or die, you have been given a gift of unique power. Anyone who was touched by your ordeal, whether very close to you or at the outer circles in turn must value their own lives—the brief time we have on this earth—with much greater intensity, and a far greater imperative simply to praise the One who brought us here. The thankfulness to God with which you used to fall asleep each night must for you personally be increased a thousandfold. But knowledge of your story has had the same effect on those who know it ... from the Latin translation of the Gospel of John, Lux in tenebris lucet et tenebrae eam non comprehenderunt. *"The light shines in the darkness and the darkness has not overcome (or encompassed, or understood) it."*

You write about the awe you felt when you learned of how many people, even people who barely know you or did not know you at all, had been praying for you. That means they were asking God, or however they understood God, to let you live. To spare your life. And the impression one gets from reading your words is that, in addition to whatever deepest resources you brought to bear in your struggle to life even while comatose, and in addition to whatever medical miracles the doctors were able to work, God heard those prayers and was moved by them. They helped. They worked.

I personally do not believe that, had your life not been spared, we should conclude that "prayer does not work." Many have prayed and not been delivered from their distress. God's mercy is different than that. But prayer does connect us ... to a power greater than ourselves, and lays before that power our deepest fears and desires. Prayer is a kind of sacrifice or offering: We bring our very hearts to the Creator and lay them before Him. We ask Him to hear us. Linear time does not matter to God, and so He has all eternity to hear the prayers of a pilot as his burning plane plunges into the sea. Prayer makes us fully human—in other words, helps us to remember who we really are: children of the Lord Most High, sons and daughters of the King, individually cherished and beloved.

In your case, what happened (who knows what happened?) is that these concentric circles of those who loved or cared about you, or were simply moved by your plight, made their voices heard to God and opened their hearts to Him, thus joining their hearts to His mighty heart. And He heard those prayers with an infinite and tender love, the "Love that moves the sun and all the other stars," as Dante wrote. The endless flow of those prayers for you and His outpouring of love in response created, I believe, a luminous tide that lifted you up off the rocks that held you in such danger. And you sailed free, and sailed home.

I want also to remind you that your very desire to live and not die was itself a kind of prayer. God says to Deuteronomy, "This day I have set before you life and death. Therefore choose life." And you did. And that is a prayer in itself, a prayer of praise ...

It has been a privilege to know you.

With love,

Kimberly

On my first day back to work, I took my seat on the 5:50 AM bus, just like old times, when I heard a voice from behind.

"You're back!"

I turned to see a pleasant fellow whose face was familiar to me only from the commute. "Yes, and glad to be back," I said. "How did you know?"

"From the bus stop," he said. "We all knew. We were all praying for you."

I didn't even know his name.

◆ ◆ ◆

As one might have expected, everything in my life was ratcheted up, my physical senses and also my spiritual. This included church. The services often bordered on the exquisite in the setting of the simple and elegant old meetinghouse that was the church's home, with the chosen music, and, of course, Harold's sermons. One he delivered a few months after my return had special resonance:

October 18, 1998

Sheer Mortality

Doesn't everything die at last, and too soon?

—Mary Oliver

Let's cut right to the chase. Autumn is a difficult time of year for many of us, including me. The summer is gone, it's over, and the beauty of early autumn serves mainly as a reminder of what we have lost ... Autumn feels like moving on to somewhere else, never stasis or status quo ...

That's not a bad thing, of course. For I need to be reminded of the passage of my time and the shortness of my days. And if it takes a cold, gray day in autumn to do that, well, so be it. If it is true, as Franz Kafka wrote, that "the meaning of life is that it ends," then I need to be reminded.

... for poet Mary Oliver, it is a "summer day" that leads to ultimate questions:

Doesn't everything die at last, and too soon?
Tell me, what is it you plan to do
With your one wild and precious life?

Given death, what shall I do with my life? According to my colleague Forrester Church, it's the most important religious question of all, for religion, he says, is nothing more than "our human response to the dual reality of being alive and having to die."

And what if, as Kafka implies, it is death that gives life its meaning, that gives our lives their meanings? Can it possibly be true?

Chaim Potok suggests it in his novel, My Name Is Asher Lev. *The protagonist, Asher Lev, remembers "the way my father looked at a bird lying on its side against the curb near our house:"*

"Is it dead, Papa?" I was six and could not bring myself to look at it.

"Yes," I heard him say in a sad and distant way.

"Why did it die?"

"Everything that lives must die."

"Everything?"

"Yes."

"You too, Papa? And Mama?"

"Yes."

"And me?"

"Yes," he said. Then he added in Yiddish, "But may it be only after you live a long and good life, my Asher."

I could not grasp it. I forced myself to look at the bird.

Everything alive would one day be as still as that bird?

"Why?" I asked.

"That's the way the Robbono Shel Olom made His world, Asher."

"Why?"

"So life would be precious, Asher. Something that is yours forever is never precious."

Obvious as it seems, there are too many people in the world who just don't seem to get it ...

Unfortunately, many religions ask us to deny our mortality: to deny the very thing that gives our lives their meaning. They ask us to ignore the reality of death, to look away, and to hope for some better life than the one we have been miraculously given, the one which is already ours.

To look away from death is, I believe, to refuse to take life seriously. Ernest Morgan, who has written a good deal about death, writes that:

Suddenly, as you face the reality of your own death, familiar things around you explode into vivid interest and meaning. The shape of that leaf, the color of that rock, the movement of that cloud has something to say to you. You become hungry for knowledge about the plants and animals of this strange planet on which you briefly find yourself. Life becomes fresh and exciting. How can a person be bored, waste time, or think petty thoughts in the midst of such an experience? With no time to lose, one must develop the quality of his life to the utmost. Only in lively and intense commitment can the greatest satisfaction be found …

One cannot help but wonder if in this most horrendous century of violence and bloodshed, we have somehow forgotten the preciousness of life in the face of death: We take life so lightly that it is all too easy to deny our shared mortality.

I'm talking about sheer *mortality. For we are always standing on the brink, though we would rather not think about it. But the point is, we* must *think about it if we are to become the better people we wish to be. In the face of his own impending death, Mitch Albom's friend Morrie [in his book* Tuesdays With Morrie*] has some suggestions for how to live. They are sensible and simple:*

Be compassionate … and take responsibility for each other.
Love each other or die.
Forgive yourself before you die. Then forgive others.
You need to make peace with yourself and everyone around you.

The important questions, he says, "… have to do with love, responsibility, spirituality, awareness. And if I were healthy today, those would still be my issues. They should have been all along.

"Devote yourself to loving others, devote yourself to your community around you, and devote yourself to creating something that gives you purpose and meaning." *As a kind of summary of what death has taught him, Morris says,* "Love is the only rational act …"

So, if someone asks you if you are a religious person, take a look at your commitments. You may be surprised to find just how "religious" you are or (and there is value in this discovery as well) just how religious you aren't.

Which bring us back to that pressing question posed by the recognition of our sheer mortality: What shall I do with my life? Only you can decide! Only you can determine how religious your life is going to be. But you had better decide, for as Amiel writes, "Life is short, and we never have too much time to gladden the hearts of those traveling the dark journey with us. O, be swift to love, make haste to be kind."

Time hastens onward, and autumn reminds me of that. If, as Mary Oliver suggests, prayer is paying attention, then let us pray that we never take our lives too lightly. May we be always attentive to ourselves, to those around us, and to the earth our home. May we be guided by love. And let us pay particular attention to the reality of life's ending. For though that ending ever be "too soon," it ultimately is what gives our lives their meaning.

> "Tell me, what is it you plan to do
> With your one wild and precious life?"
> —Mary Oliver

The greatest miracle is the discovery that all is miraculous. And the nature of the miraculous is—utter simplicity.

—Henry Miller

Epilogue One

For more than two years following my discharge from Spaulding Rehab, I enjoyed a near miraculous recovery. After regaining my initial strength through swimming and outpatient physical therapy, I resumed my former, active lifestyle. I went back to work at John Hancock, returned to the tennis court, worked out at the gym, and even cross-country skied to mountaintops in Vermont and sailed with B.G. Most important of all, I was able to return to being a fun, active mom for Westy and Lindsay, which was a huge relief for their dad.

My most troublesome physical symptoms during this time were a stiffness in my legs that would come on after some amount of exertion and a greater level of daily fatigue than before. My short-term memory was also greatly affected, but I have developed several coping mechanisms, such as making copious notes, that enable me to navigate daily life with some degree of success.

After an early scare following my illness, Dr. Scammell once explained that because my central nervous system was beaten up so badly by ADEM, "anything could happen." He compared my nervous system to a "patched together electrical system." In the fall of 2000, something did happen. After a respiratory flu weakened my system, the neuromuscular symptoms in my legs returned, and they never went away. That is when the doctors gave me a diagnosis of multiple sclerosis (MS), something I thought that I had evaded. When this stunning diagnosis came down, with all of its terrible uncertainty, I was in disbelief, perhaps even a bit of shock. I thought that because I had been doing so well, perhaps the diagnosis would turn out to be wrong. But the symptoms persist and are with me always.

Despite the stiffness and weakness in my legs, my situation has remained fairly stable. As of this writing, I can still walk without a device. I just can't be on my feet for any length of time without my legs aching. I may no longer be able to terrorize Bruce on the tennis court, but I row nearly every summer day that I can, which I love. Perhaps if I could still play tennis, I might not have discovered this new joy. I also have my sight and the complete function of my upper body. Most importantly, I can still care for my children.

Several people from the medical community have voiced their belief that there will be a cure for MS in my lifetime. One can certainly hope, and I do hope that medical research will be able to move forward on this and so many other debilitating diseases. Meanwhile, I count myself as one of the lucky ones. Symptoms of MS fall across a wide spectrum, and I know, once again, that I have been blessed.

Epilogue Two

In October 2007, Bruce received a diagnosis of a rare and deadly cancer. It quickly proved to be inoperable, but he responded well to chemotherapy for several months. Watching this strong, vibrant, handsome person fade away before our eyes was my second crucible. He died in July 2008. I had dreaded his being in despair, as he would have to understand his dreadful prognosis: the aggressive cholangocarcinoma. But he was truly amazing. He was so strong and constructive, even taking vitamins in hospice! His positive outlook and nobility filled us with awe. He still made us laugh, even to the end.

His desire for normalcy set his family strongly down a path of carrying on, doing well, and enjoying life, which I know will continue to serve us well. I can only hope that our magnificent children are doing as well as it seems. They are so stoic that it may be hard to tell. But they are doing well in school and having happy times with nice friends. That is all I hope for.

We still can't believe that B.G. is gone, but at least we had him for a while—for a wondrous, fun, lovely while.

He was our shooting star.

My Magnificent Hospitals

It is my great hope that this story might inspire people who are so moved to make contributions to Beth Israel Deaconess Medical Center, their Neurology Education and Research Fund, or to Spaulding Rehabilitation Hospital.

These superlative institutions—both Harvard Medical School teaching hospitals—are located in Boston, and private contributions enable them to continue their research and to care for patients in need.

I will be forever indebted to these hospitals, and to their doctors, nurses and therapists, first for persevering to save my life, and then for enabling me to reclaim my life.

Beth Israel Deaconess Medical Center
c/o Development Department
330 Brookline Avenue
Boston, Massachusetts 02215

BIDMC Neurology Education and Research Fund
330 Brookline Avenue
Boston, Massachusetts 02215

Spaulding Rehabilitation Hospital
c/o Development Department
125 Nashua Street
Boston, Massachusetts 02214

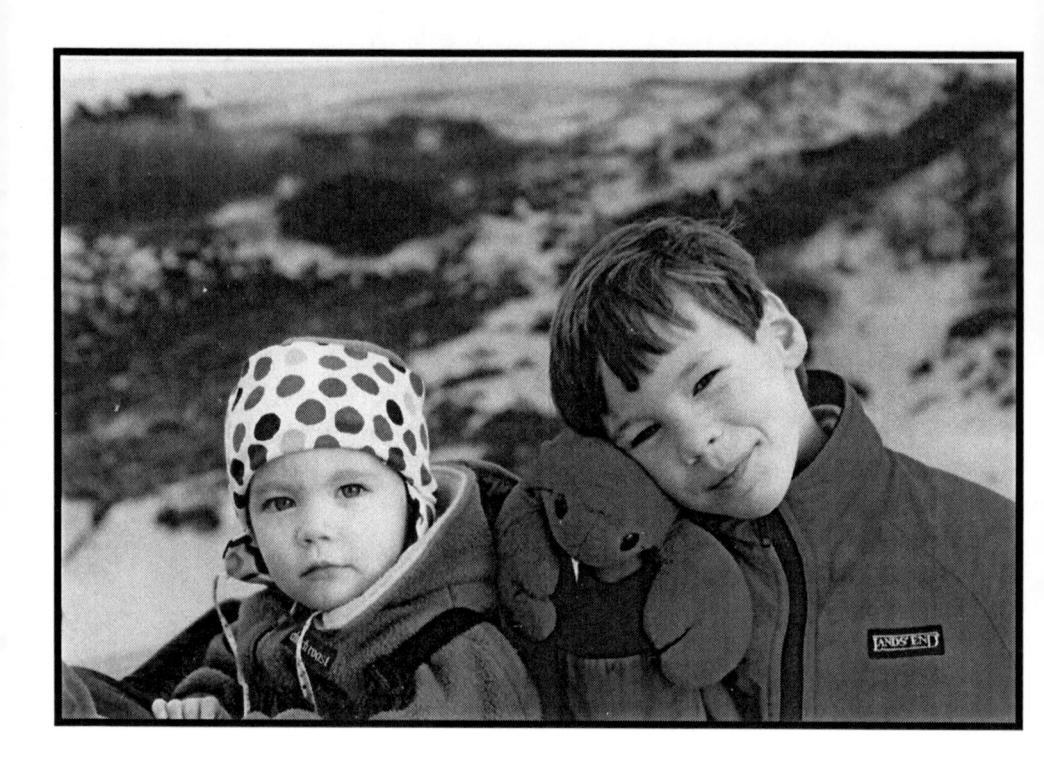

This is the photograph of our children that Bruce brought for me. It was at my bedside at the MICU at Beth Israel-Deaconess and at Spaulding Rehab. It meant so much to me to be able to look at my children and remind myself of the main reason for getting well. When I might have thought that I couldn't possibly work any harder, looking at this beautiful picture of Westy and Lindsay reminded me that no amount of work and exhaustion was too much—if I could only get back home.

Acknowledgments

I am indebted to the doctors who not only saved my life and helped me regain my lost abilities, but who then took their time and energy to help illuminate medical information and offer moving insights and dramatic observations of my case.

Their encouragement and support was deeply moving, and I felt extraordinarily privileged to benefit from their interest, time, and willingness to help. I thank Dr. Thomas Scammell, who headed my neurology team at the Beth Israel-Deaconess Medical Center in Boston (BIDMC) and is Assistant Professor of Neurology, Harvard Medical School; Dr. Joel Stein, Director of Stroke Rehabilitation and the Chief Medical Officer at Spaulding Rehabilitation Hospital (SRH) in Boston, and Assistant Professor of Physical Medicine, Harvard Medical School; Dr. David Trentham, a rheumatologist at BIDMC; and Dr. Paul Sandhu and Dr. Adam Agranoff Harvard Medical School resident fellows at Massachusetts General Hospital and SRH.

Judy Atterstrom, my primary nurse at BIDMC's medical intensive care unit, also spoke at length with me as I tried to recapture the missing spaces in my memory from the time I became comatose. I conducted a weekslong interview with Teresa McLaughlin, my primary nurse at SRH. My lead physical therapist at SRH, Dawn Lucier, also contributed her insights and helped me decipher the mysteries of physical therapy shorthand in the SRH progress notes.

Professor Kimberley Patton, Marisa Morin, and Laurie Burlingame generously provided enlightenment in their respective areas of expertise. The Reverend Harold Babcock, of the First Religious Society, Unitarian Universalist, in Newburyport, Massachusetts, graciously gave permission to excerpt one of his sermons. Sheridan McCarthy, my iUniverse editor, provided invaluable guidance, encouragement and understanding in helping me prepare this book for publication.

In addition to the doctors, nurses, and therapists, my loved ones—family and friends—also revisited this emotionally trying time to help me put together the pieces of a lost chapter of my life. My brother Kim Chapin provided invaluable editorial guidance. I am most grateful to my husband, Bruce, and my mother, Roberta Chapin, for reaching back into a nightmare.

Spring 1998 was undoubtedly more difficult for them than anyone could begin to imagine.

I hope that I have done the story justice, with its many heroics and victories, and the pervasive generosity and human kindness at its core. So many, near and far, both familiar and unknown to me, helped me and my family during a terrible time, and we shall never forget.

Notes

1. Increased fluid in tissues that accompanies inflammation, such as the swelling of a bee sting. A T2 image is a type of MRI scan used to indicate areas of edema, with or without swelling. Increased or decreased T2 signal on the MRI, depending on whether the area looks white or blacker than normal, also referred to as hyperintensity or hypointensity, respectively.

2. Infections break down cells, whose proteins are then discharged into the spinal fluid, as revealed in a spinal tap. But an acute demyelinating process would produce the same result in a spinal tap. Demyelination is the destruction of the myelin sheath that insulates the axon, the portion of the nerve cells that acts as both insulation and conduit.

3. Medical note: Lumbar puncture should be performed as early as possible in patients suspected of having ADEM because other more life-threatening illnesses may be part of the differential diagnosis in the initial phase of the disease. The diagnosis of bacterial meningitis with secondary vascular insult, viral meningoencephalitis, and even cerebral or cord hemorrhages must be strongly considered.
—"Acute Disseminated Encephalomyelitis: A Case-Based Review" by Ramsis Benjamin, MD, and Gregory Y. Chang, MD, *Hospital Physician,* November 1998

4. A micro-organism that causes typhus and other typhus-like fevers.

5. Laurie Burlingame, a young friend of ours who was studying neuroscience at Harvard Medical School, wrote this explanation of the role that myelin played within the central nervous system and why, in my case, its destruction was so devastating. It also helped me understand why a diagnosis was so difficult. As I later read her essay, I kept in mind the two essential points. The axon was essentially a conduit along which impulses travel from one nerve cell to the next, and myelin was an insulating material that surrounded the axon.

   Myelin, which is produced from within the central nervous system, is an insulating material that surrounds, or ensheathes, the axon so that nerve impulses can travel quickly and efficiently from one part of the body to another. These nerve impulses are called action potentials. They are created when a neuron in one cell reaches a threshold value. They then travel along the axon to the next nerve cell. Once this action potential reaches the end of the axon, a process occurs that causes this impulse to bind to the next neuron, generating a response. This response can be one of many things.

The key is that the successful passage of the action potential down the length of the axon is essential for all neural communication, which in turn is central to the development of virtually every kind of behavioral response, whether it is a muscle contraction, the ability to see, or the ability to solve a complex math problem.

This action potential is made up of positively charged ions that move along the axon much like electricity. And, much like electricity, these ions will take the path of least resistance and try to flow out of the axon altogether. When myelin is present to insulate the axon, the path of least resistance for the ions is down the center of the axon.

Myelin also helps speed up the delivery of action potentials. This is because myelin does not run the entire length of the axon, but gathers in many conglomerations, in between which are unmyelinated nodes, known as the nodes of Raviner. At these nodes of Raviner, the action potential is passed along to the next myelinated part of the axon. In this way, the action potential appears to skip down the axon, a process known as saltatory conduction. But if there is no myelin, the ions responsible for passing along the action potentials will leave the axon. Thus, the signal many never reach its destination—the synaptic button at the beginning of the next nerve cell.

Many of the components of the myelin sheath are immune proteins. Demyelination occurs when, for reasons not clearly understood, the immune system misfunctions and begins to attack proteins that it once recognized as belonging to the self as if they were foreign invaders: bacteria, for example.

The immune system has a variety of ways to destroy molecules that are not seen as the self. One way is to secrete harmful chemicals that destroy protein. When demyelination occurs, it interferes with salatory conduction—the passing along of the action potentials. The result is that action potentials now are passed along very slowly, and may never reach their destination at all. This is detrimental. Without the arrival of a particular action potential, a chain of events leading to a particular kind of behavior cannot take place. For example, individuals with multiple sclerosis have a lack of coordination, overall weakness, and impaired vision and speech.

The rate of return of myelin is extremely slow and in some cases does not occur at all. Again, this is something that is poorly understood.

About the Cover Art

Susan Murray Stokes, a Copley Master Portraitist, born in England and now living in Newbury, Massachusetts, is a dear friend who asked me to sit for her. This illustration was made the year before my illness. Susan made the sketch in about one hour's time. I love sitting for Susan and having the time to visit with her. On that day, I was literally watching Lindsay, then a toddler, as she played on the floor of Susan's studio. I think the image is one of true motherhood and somewhat evocative, perhaps the calm hinting of the storm to come.

In the early days at Spaulding Rehab, when I came to understand what had happened to me, one of the first things I remembered was finally having had the sketch framed and hanging it on the wall in Lindsay's nursery only weeks before I became ill. I was so grateful to Susan, knowing that Lindsay had an image to remind her of her mother every day, during my long time away from her and Westy that year.

Wendy Chapin Ford

June 2009

Computer graphics courtesy of Westy Ford

Breinigsville, PA USA
21 January 2010

231123BV00001B/19/P